Come Jog With Me

George D. Whitney, DVM

Come Jog With Me

iUniverse books may be ordered through booksellers or by contacting:

iUniverse
1663 Liberty Drive
Bloomington, IN 47403
www.iuniverse.com
1-800-Authors (1-800-288-4677)

Layout and design provided by
Howard Printing, Inc.
Brattleboro, Vermont

Certain stock imagery © Th inkstock.

ISBN: 978-1-4620-7300-9 (sc)
ISBN: 978-1-4620-7302-3 (hc)
ISBN: 978-1-4620-7301-6 (e)

Printed in the United States of America

iUniverse rev. date: 12/20/2011

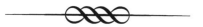

*For President
Barack and
Michelle Obama*

*The two brightest
stars on the horizon*

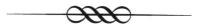

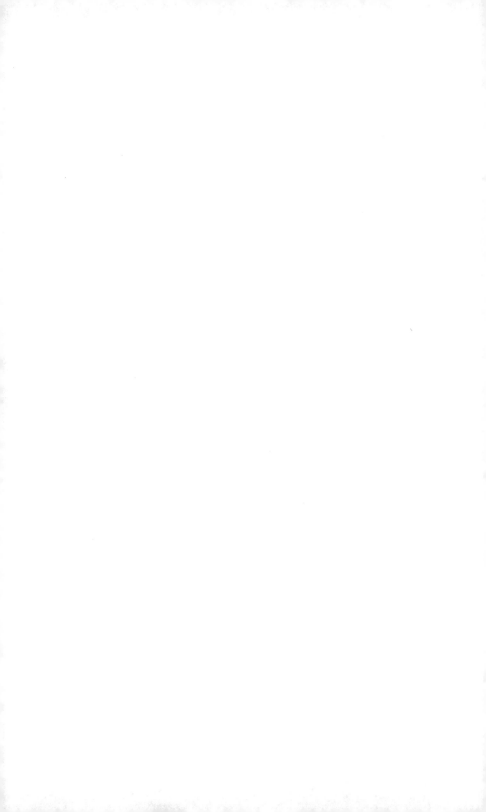

An Open Letter to President Barack Obama

Dear President Obama,

This book is dedicated to you and Mrs. Obama for many reasons among which is both of your dedication to efforts of better health for all. The significance of my thesis of the importance of running type exercise should not be underestimated. As you may know runners rarely have strokes. Strokes are listed as one of the top three causes of death. Strokes cost in the neighborhood of $250,000 for each case treated in the hospital.

An insurance figure for 2007 reported that 750,000 elderly people were admitted to hospitals in our country from falls around the house. We know runners rarely have fractures from falling and the cost of care for those 750,000 hospital cases has to be astronomical. I read that women runners have as much as half the incidence of breast cancer as non-running women.

My message is that runners are so much healthier than non-exercisers. They need only a fraction of the medical costs as non-runners. I hope my book has enough common sense for seniors to start a craze of running for health reasons as well as for the fun of it that will, incidentally, reduce the cost of medical care appreciably.

This book points to evidence that problems such as

Autism in children and in canines, Hip Dysplasia, are from toxins in diets and not from the Zebra causes so many scientists are searching for without success.

Please accept my best wishes and appreciation of your efforts for all and "Illegitimi non carborundum."

George Whitney, DVM

An Open Letter to Mrs. Michelle Obama

Dear Mrs. Obama,

Your efforts on behalf of children are exciting and important. Having undertaken the process of becoming a student of running, I have a suggestion the implementation of which could have profound desirable effects on children in our time but also on the health of the general population in the future.

You are aware of the overwhelming evidence of better health in those who exercise regularly over non-exercisers. Moreover it is accepted that those who learn to exercise early in life are more apt to continue.

Observing students at recess periods there are those who enter into physical activities and other children who avoid such when all able children should enter them. A suggestion of starting all able children on the exercise of running from pre-school age and through high school is an idea that could yield remarkable results at no additional cost to the school board.

Orange cones used by most highway departments could be available for all to be used during recess periods in mornings and afternoons most schools provide. The cones would be placed at appropriate distances apart for each aged child group to run around. Some might require adults to hand hold the tiny tots while learning.

By high school, talent would be discovered that would keep many potential dropouts running on the school track team.

With over 30,000,000* estimated to run at least once a week in our country, the results of early learning could result in another 30,000,000 joining the good health of the first with a remarkable financial savings in medical services and medication from better health.

It is also my hope that after considering the objectives of this book you might enter the running mystique for the good of yourself and loved ones.

With Respect and Ultimate Admiration,

George Whitney

George Whitney, DVM

---

* USA Track and Field

Preface

It is estimated that at least 30 million people in our country run at least once a week.* Having started when 80 years of age, I have relearned to run as all had done as children. Now after almost 11 years of running in organized races for my health as well as for fun, I have gained knowledge to share with the millions of non-runners of our land for their good as well as for fun.

My initial reason for this book was to show by example how I did it and to attempt to convince the millions of non-runners that, first, they have the inherited ability to run and, second, to convince all inactive, over-65-years-of-age people to join me. I am told repeatedly that my attempt will be a failure because so many have convinced themselves that running is work and as senior years pass the object is to enjoy rest and inactivity.

In studying the approach to being convincing led to a surprising number of conclusions that may be nothing less than astounding when analyzed for a road to better health.

Questions in life flow like a river with many questions having less than satisfactory answers. This book presents theories for answers and I expect the readers will evaluate each answer to questions such as: Why do so many people run regularly? Can all normal people of any age relearn to

* USA Track and Field

run? Why are runners said to be healthier than non-runners? Why do runners live longer than non-runners? Why do running women have so much less incidence of breast cancer than non-running women? Why are running and jogging fun? Why have humans inherited the ability to run? Why are those who exercise most considered the healthiest? How could the cost of health care be reduced by at least 50 percent by non-runners learning to run? How could man's best friend have influenced all of us to have the running capability? Finally, why should humans be considered a dog's best friend?

All of these questions are answered in *Come Jog With Me* and many more.

The chapters are called "Laps" because I did most of my relearning on running tracks of Yale University and I coin the word, "TIE," an acronym for "take it easy," to encourage new senior runners to TIE.

It has been said that there have been books that have actually changed history, one such was *Uncle Tom's Cabin* that helped to abolish slavery and another is *The Jungle* that resulted in cleaning up the packing house scandals and proved the value of unions and food hygiene.

I believe this book may be such a book and here are some reasons. More and more evidence indicates exercise as intense as running as part of human living is necessary for the healthiest life as we interpret it. Why humans inherit the ability to run distances and those who run are so much healthier than non-runners, when appreciated and accepted can result in positive lifestyle changes for all healthy non-running humans who accept the challenge in this book.

Science accepts the fact that part of human life is dependent on the removal of waste products in human metabolism. I have not heard of science addressing the need of the exercise produced by running to be perhaps a necessary part of optimal exercise. The suggestion I pose is that running exercise results in much greater passage of blood through the detoxifying organs such as the liver, kidneys, spleen, and lymph system, etc., than happens with most other exercise. The actual pounding of the feet on the pavement for periods may enhance the ability of the internal organs to flush out the wastes that most other exercise is incapable of.

Scientists are delving into the functions of the brain as never before in history. Reports of chemical changes in our brains that have profound influences in our well being have been mentioned. It may be that the slight jarring of the brain with each running step aids in the favorable brain chemistry that other exercises do not equal.

Acknowledgements

To my late wife, Dorothy, who was supportive in many of my activities including, at the time, my new interest in running and then encouraging me to write about it for others to enjoy, I am forever grateful. To my daughter, Lee, who typed three complete revisions and later, hours of correcting the last manuscript as well as having better things to do with her busy schedule including watching over me, I am grateful. To my computer coach son, Chuck who at the time of my considering running was a teacher and track coach of the Ellsworth High School track team in Ellsworth, Maine, and himself a distance runner. To my daughter, Kate, who has given support and transportation to many races. To Coach Chuck's daughter and my granddaughter, Beth Whitney, who contributed the picture on the cover of this book of me half way on a winter's 5k race. To my "on location" coach, Chris Dickerson, a class runner and friend who was ever handy to talk with about the sport and make suggestions. To high school coach and teacher, Joe Steel, who not only gave me support but supplied me with countless memorable photographs, as did John Grant, Richard Nelson and countless other photo takers. I have mentioned the three major race directors in the text and others such as Tom Kulhawik, a runner himself who is the official timer of many Connecticut races and Ed Snyder, MD, who seemed concerned with my efforts and regularly met me with a shoulder and water after many races in which we both ran. To Richard Zbrozek, who may hold the record for the largest number of races he runs in, in any of recent years has been supportive and interesting to talk with about the sport. To columnist Randy Beach who has reported on my activities over the years. After daughter Lee and I had been the only ones to read the manuscript, I asked trophy- winning runner and linguist Bob Stephenson to read it and offer any suggestions. He mentioned that perhaps I should have spent more pages on just the jogging rather than the organized racing. Being a true story, I believe many of those who try the jogging will enjoy it so much it will evolve to running in races as it did for me. Time will tell. Thanks also to Howard Printing (particularly Ben Briggs and Donna McElligott) here in Brattleboro, Vermont, for putting so many pieces of the late drafts together before printing. To all mentioned and so many other supporters, I hereby give thanks.

Contents

Lap 1 ~ The Revelation

In the "Solace for All Retirement Home" a group of senior residents have gathered in a lounge. It's a pleasant sunny room with old folks talking about the weather and the television is on with a couple watching. Two women are playing Scrabble, two others are knitting, others are sitting. One of the men winks at a woman across the room and she winks back. Shortly the two stand up and walk to a hallway. Someone comments, "I wonder where they're going?" The couple walks briskly to and up the staircase. Shortly they come down the stairs with bright colored running shorts on, different colored socks, running shoes and "T" shirts, one with "CALL 911" on it and the other, "RUN FOR YOUR LIFE." They jog out of the doorway and down the walk to the road and are seen jogging out of sight. When the man winked to his friend he was signaling, "Come Jog with Me" and her return wink said, "Let's go!"

I want you to know that most (65 year olds and up) are capable of getting in shape to be able to run for the fun of it as well as for the good of it. This is my plea for you to do the same. It is because of the wonderful change in my life that I want you to know you also can enjoy the fun of running as I have. As a very young man I had enjoyed a little jogging and running but from high school days on I was not inclined to run or even to scamper very much. However at age 80 I jogged 100 yards or so to our mailbox and nearly collapsed. It was a rude awakening and as I walked slowly home I wondered if my heart was failing. It was obvious that something was very wrong with me. Son, Chuck, was a high school track coach at the Ellsworth, Maine, High School and I contacted him for a program to attempt to "get in shape." The following is an uncomplicated "how I did it" and how you can do it and enjoy the fun with the effort.

You dedicate an hour a day, 3 times a week to "getting in shape." Perhaps Monday, Wednesday and Friday at 7 AM. In the beginning you do not use up the entire hour until you are able.

Your first walk must not be too tiring. Simple? It's as simple as that BUT you must dedicate yourself to 3 times a week. It depends on you to discover how long it takes you to be able to walk for an hour. When you accomplish that hour's walk you have reached an important point in your adventure because it is at that point that the next "step" can be taken. You may say, "I can walk for an hour right now." Fine, you are ready for the first stride of a jog right now.

As you walk you decide to jog if even for only 6 to 10 paces and return to your walk. You are the only one who knows when you tire from the few jogging paces so you make your own decision. Increase the jogging time in your walk until you are alternating jogging with as many paces as you are walking. It may be quite suddenly that you feel an unexpected pleasure with no ill effects in those few first paces of jogging. Furthermore every time you find you can increase the jogging it becomes more and more satisfying. Soon you will return from your hour's walking and jogging feeling so elated about your improvement that you will be overjoyed. This process must be a gradual one until you can jog for that hour even if your jogging is slow. This may take a year. Eureka, you are a runner.

From experience I learned that although progress becomes obvious and fun you may have the tendency to overdo. So I have found the word, "TIE" is a good one to remember and it stands for "Take It Easy." For me, I was so elated in my progress at about 6 months of the program that I did not TIE and became too stiff after an hour's effort. Still, by the time a year was up I was able to jog, if only in one place, for an hour. That was another special time in my adventure. I discovered I could jog for an hour three times a week and was proud of myself. As I passed my 81st birthday, I wondered about scheduled organized races I had heard about.

For a little added incentive to get started, try to contact a running club or store or even one runner in your area and ask for a volunteer to join you and friends who want to try to put the advice in this book to work. Running stores will either send one of their employees or another runner who will gladly join you for a few early attempts to get started. With each of those contacts, you will be introduced to the strange enthusiasm of the established runner who will enjoy your experience him or herself.

Somewhere along the line of embracing the thought of jogging you should ask your doctor's permission to try running.* In passing your physical exam you may have accomplished an extra plus. Among your test results there may be a couple of tests showing that, although normal, you are low normal. If, in the future you have to go for another exam for a problem, your low normal findings on record then will be considered normal for you and not misleading a diagnosis.

Don't let minor problems dissuade you from at least trying my program and don't let minor injuries occurring along the way discourage you either.

There is more and more evidence that for painful knees and other joints, running may be the answer by stimulating healing of problems but in the last analysis let you and your doctor make that decision as to running. I do have anatomical problems. But I have absolutely no pains anywhere at this time.

*Appendix 1, page 148

Lap 2 ~ Get Set and Go for It

Next comes a period of well-meaning friends and jealous onlookers trying to discourage you, but hopefully you are dedicated to at least trying your hand, or I should say feet, at actually running. In my case it was for several months of slow jogging for an hour that were not only easy but enjoyable and my heart had held up.

If you have decided to attempt to break the shackles that keep you from utilizing your physical potential, the above is one proven way to do it. If so, you may consider the next step that I call your insurance policy explained in Lap 5.

Many friends had mentioned that running would ruin my knees. At one point I decided that was a prophetic observation. About two months into the early jogging, my 80-year-old left knee became painful resulting in a limp while walking. I contacted my Coach who told me to keep on the schedule but make the workouts much lighter. In a few weeks my left knee was less painful but the right knee was painful. In several more weeks both knees were normal. Since, after over 5,000 miles of running in training and racing, I have had no discomfort in either knee.

The internet became more active as the Coach's advice in the communications was frequent. I suspect at this point Coach Chuck thought, "I think the old man may be serious." Indeed I had become more serious.

If you do join the action even for a trial period and even if it's only to get into some kind of shape, you should consider keeping a log. As you walk and then jog a little, keep the log in mind and after every session enter what you might want to refer to later on. I keep track of the distance during each episode and sometimes the time too. Weather and temperature may be of interest. In preparation of turning a page of the log book, I note the total miles recorded and carry it forward to the next page. In my case, for example, as I said, since I started to keep track in 1999, I have logged over 5,000 miles. They do add up. How far is it across our land?

When you reach the racing stage the results are published promptly after every race on the computer and they include a list of the runners, your position among the finishers, your time and the speed per mile. For some races I wish my record was not recorded. I am told the editors of *Running Times Magazine* will send you a free log book if requested. *

* See Appendix 8, page 164

Lap 3 ~ An Inspiration?

Having come this far in the reading if not in the actual activity and being of average intelligence or better, you may consider dipping a toe in the water to test the temperature. Just give jogging a try. Nothing ventured, nothing gained. Look in the back of a closet for a pair of old sneakers and put them on and with appropriate other clothing go out by yourself, because at your age you don't want to look foolish to your friends unless the cause is great enough. Try my formula. If you do it, in a short while you won't give a damn what others think because you will feel so great you may consider continuing as I have done and then you may be elated enough to write a book. Your grandchildren will delight in telling their friends, "My Grand-father (or mother) runs for a hobby."

The reason for the above is because that is the way I felt when I began. I felt the same at my first race and also embar-rassed. In order to make light of my racing effort, I printed some slogans on the backs of a few shirts. One coach sug-gested, "OXYGEN IS OVERRATED" and the other, "RUN-NING FROM THE UNDERTAKER." Many runners were distracted over my incompetence as a runner by the humor of the slogans. I now have a collection of over 100 shirts with my homemade, mostly plagiarized slogans that have added many smiles that would otherwise not have been present on earth.*

* See Appendix 6, page 155

The object of this book is to get men and women off their butts and out improving themselves. If you are a senior citizen, whatever age that may be, and start running I will guarantee at races there will be those who will look you in the eye and say, "You are an inspiration."

I predict that the time is fast approaching when your physician will tell you, man or woman, the time has come for you to take medication to control heart and blood vessel problems and then he or she will say, "Of course there is an alternative and that is to take up running as therapy." Better to do it before you need pills as a therapy.

Lap 4 ~ Why Humans Run

Not being satisfied with the variety of answers to the questions, "Why do so many humans run?" and "Why doesn't everybody run?" I hereby propose an answer. Just as our ancestors developed the ability with the anatomy to be able to run for distances so I conclude we inherited a subconscious desire to run. The question immediately arises, "Why, then don't all people run?" The answer to that involves the tendency to avoid work and our subconscious tells us that running is not only work but hard work. We are told at an early age that we should do everything and anything to get out of work. The electric toothbrush is an example. We are inundated with technology to get out of work that overrides the subconscious for many but not for the 30 million of us who do run at least once a week. Much technology is welcome and useful.

Many of our customs discourage exercise such as high heels and clothing in vogue which discourages it. The suggestion, "That seems like work to me." Seems to be an indelible statement in our language. So in effect the reason runners hesitate before answering that question may be because they don't actually know why. However, the reasons for continuing to feel better and to keep in shape and a dozen others are the convenient and common answers.

For many runners the thought of stopping their running is to accept a black ticket on the train of life.

Lap 5 ~ An Insurance Policy

Years ago my elders gave me the impression that I should leave this world better than I have found it. Surely that is why I am in a position to write this book. It has to be because others left this world better than they found it. To get down to the actual reason for this effort, it is to sell you a free insurance policy. Yes, I mean to verbally "sell." I mean to sell an idea with the expectations that you will buy.

Even if you are one of so many mature men and women who when asked if they ever considered running for the fun of it have answered something like this, "Run? That is without a doubt the last thing I would ever have even thought about." If you are in that category, you are one I will try to sell my free policy to. If you are in the following categories I want to sell you insurance too. It would ruin my knees or it's too much like work or my husband (wife) wouldn't let me or I'm afraid of dogs chasing me or no time and on and on come the excuses.

If you are interested in the provisions of the free insurance policy how would the following provisions seem to you?

1. Rarely insomnia
2. Loss of weight
3. Feeling of euphoria
4. Becoming happier

5. Becoming healthier
6. Having more comfortable feet
7. Loss of stiffness in joints
8. Easier climbing stairs
9. Easier to get along with
10. Fewer cerebral accidents (strokes)
11. Less coronary artery disease
12. Less atherosclerosis
13. Few have Alzheimer's Disease
14. You will have bragging rights for your children, grandchildren and perhaps even for your great-grandchildren
15. Stronger bones
16. Later onset of diabetes by years
17. Few pills to take

I should hasten to note all the above may not relate to you and also that there are many other and perhaps minor pluses such as living an average of two or more years longer than non-runners. If you do accept my policy it means you have gained wisdom that may have taken 65 years to acquire. In my case it took me 80 years to appreciate that wisdom.

In offering my insurance policy I can point out an overweight elderly woman who is having trouble walking and I can say that with my policy, embraced and adopted a few years previously she would be walking with ease today. The chances are that she would weigh less, and human physicians report regularly that women who run have better bone density than others. Pages could be filled with examples such as runners rarely die of strokes, runners have lower blood pressure and more good cholesterol than non-runners and so on.

Woven into my prescription and insurance policy is the story of my adventure. For you to benefit as I have, you must start as I repeatedly mention with the dedication of three times a week of walking and jogging until you are able to jog for the exercise period before your next defining moment of slow running.

Don't let anyone convince you that you cannot at least try to join the action. A quote by Oliver Wendell Holmes I have used on my stationery is, "...a man...should share the action and passion of his time, at peril of being judged not to have lived." An approximate quote and can be adjusted for women.

Lap 6 ~ The Initiation

The next logical step for me was to find a real race to try out my newly developed skill. Marty Shaivonne, a race director, responded to my phone call with the location, date and a time of a race and he encouraged me to try and said, "I'll be waiting for you at the end if it takes you a week." That was the kind of comforting reply I needed. Marty was and remains a good and supporting friend. He began the recognition of older age groups in our area from, "Over 60" up to recently, "Over 90." At this point I am looking for an "Over 95" age group in a few years.

For the first race I was well advised to arrive an hour early for parking near the headquarters where there were many runners both male and female of all ages warming up. I asked one with a number pinned on his chest and was conducted to the registration desks where you pay a registration donation if you have not preregistered and get your bib which is your number for the race to pin on your front. There is usually a bag of goodies such as a sample of toothpaste, deodorant, a safety razor and notices of upcoming races, a souvenir running shirt and for me there were many, "Good Lucks."

There were introductions and with each I was told not to start too fast. With all the activity of many interested in my being a new old runner there was not time to warm up. As the starting time approached the runners started like a river to wend its way to the starting line on the road. It was a 5k race and that is 5 kilometers or 3.1 miles. At that point the director delivered a short sermon that I couldn't hear with my hearing problem. Starting at the back of the horde of runners the gun went off and everyone began jogging in place until I found myself jogging with those at the back of the pack.

It was at the first water hole one mile along that I quite suddenly realized I had been running too fast and a volunteer offered me a ride in her car to the finish line. I was mortified that my running style was obviously so bad. I declined the offer and continued where at two miles a police car pulled up alongside of me and made the same offer. I hobbled along and finished almost walking.

Finding that finish line was one of the more significant moments of my life. There was much back patting. A bottle of cold water and many using the same expression, "Nice job." Catching my breath I thought, "Eureka," an expression that would become more and more common to me. Back at the headquarters there was much laughter and applause for winners of each age and male and female category. When my name was announced as the winner of the over 80 year old group I was sure there was more applause than had been for the overall race winner. Incidentally, I was the only one in my age group.

The watermelon, in season and the variety of food and drink could satisfy anyone. On driving slowly homeward I found myself smiling in wonderment over my having accomplished something a year before I had not the slightest idea that I would ever do.

I hope readers will have the thrill of running in such a race as my first one was with the euphoria and that huge smile while driving home.

After many workouts and races I wondered why I was so pleased with myself. Then I read about a subject that seemed interesting called, "the runner's high." It may be possible and perhaps probable that the expression is more than an emotional feeling of a job well done. Has some chemical change actually taken place that is called the runner's high? At this point I am inclined to believe it has and it is a change that no couch potato will ever experience without the exercise of jogging. That seems to me to be a sad truism.

Lap 7 ~ Eureka

If because of reading this book you have finished your first race I say to you, "EUREKA and congratulations." Perhaps you are so delighted you don't need congrats because you are elated with your progress. The most important realizations deep within yourself were having done what a few months ago you could not imagine actually doing. On the way home you, too, will find yourself smiling to think of that accomplishment. As your news travels in the following days, some of those who gave you warnings may realize how wrong they were with their negative advice.

Plan to relax and give your anatomy time for a recovery for several days. You may wonder if by continuing your workouts you might shave a few minutes from that first time. After a few days rest you will again realize how well you feel, not only in your legs but in general.

It was probably about those early days I wondered about writing to older men and women who could profit and enjoy the activity as I had begun to do. Little did I recognize the health benefits for running seniors at that time.

It was also at this period I found myself looking at many non-running older and younger people too and realizing that in being able to jog that hour, three times a week, it was better than many of them could do. Along with that thought I felt invigorated. I would slap my thighs and consider how good my legs felt. Try it for yourself. Proof of the pudding.

Lap 8 ~ Second Race

With the wisdom acquired from your first race you should improve in your second. As an example, I found my second race would be almost in my backyard over trails that I had been training on. Waiting for the gun to go off, I struck up a conversation with another runner waiting as I was. He introduced himself as Chris Dickerson. After that race Chris was waiting for me with a word of encouragement. "You reduced your time by almost 10 minutes, congratulations." I was impressed that he had watched me finish the week before and was interested in my effort. Then he gave me one of the most important bits of advice I had received so far. "If you are serious about running, you should go to a running store and get fitted for a good pair of shoes and advice about the sport." That developed into my finding a group of tried and true runners who really were my introduction to the sport of running in competition. Of course competition is not necessary but it seemed like a challenging idea. Chris became my "on location" coach from then on.

Lap 9 ~ The Shoes and What's in 'Em

I took Chris's suggestion and, finding he had the only running store around, visited for more advice. There I found several qualified, proven runners to advise me about the shoes as well as many other running secrets. They had me running and walking and finally produced the "perfect" pair of shoes with the advice that if, after wearing them for a workout, they didn't feel right to return them for another pair. I learned a lot in that visit. If shoes are not right, all kinds of preventable problems can develop. If you can't wiggle your toes inside the shoes they are not right for you. If they are not right and you have a run planned out and back for a distance and develop a problem on the way out, you may have a painful walk back. The injuries are coming up shortly. Considering the cost per mile of running shoes, they are a bargain.

Overheard at one race was, "It's not the shoes but what's in 'em." I had always thought it was the reverse and investigated. In reading about the sport of running, I noticed other problems that were solved by wearing the proper shoes. Some were to prevent black toe nails, planter fasciitis (a condition of the skin of the bottom of the feet separating from the underlying tissue), weak arches, blisters, several conditions of upper legs, toeing out and in and hamstring injury. In the first place it seems to be nothing but common sense that a cushion between your feet and sometimes miles of running is better than nothing or little between your feet and the pavement.

Of course what's in the shoes is important but without proper shoes there would be far fewer runners. Even for general wear they are the most comfortable footwear ever. I used to ask people wearing running shoes if they were runners and other than at races virtually none of those questioned answered in the affirmative. The reason for running shoes for general use is obvious.

Research scientist and running expert, Professor Daniel Lieberman of Harvard, is quoted as saying, "A lot of foot and knee injuries currently plaguing us are caused by people running with shoes that actually make our feet weak, cause over pronating (ankle rotation) and give us knee problems," Perhaps low-cut inexpensive shoes are best for you.

All the information about shoes, seemed so reasonable that on asking other runners about shoes I was told that some runners swear that shoes are unnecessary. I had made up my mind so that when I found a shoeless runner at a race I questioned him. He commented on the fact that those against barefooted running have never tried it. That seemed reasonable to me and, off and on, I considered removing my shoes and different colored socks to try it. Then one day I went to the Brattleboro track to work out and there was a van with

"RUN TELLMAN, RUN" painted on it. On the track was a young bearded runner running barefooted. On questioning him he said he was preparing to run across the country from NYC to LA starting in a few weeks from then. About the bare feet he said, "Try it, you may like it." So then and there I removed my shoes and different colored socks and ran for two laps. Tellman stopped me and said that was enough or I might overdo. It was that word again, TIE. The following day the bottoms of my feet knew I had been doing something unusual. That was a fun experience I shall work on if I live that long. Tellman had feet problems and reached New Jersey without shoes. Perhaps by now shoes are a habit and on gravel or very rough surfaces I wonder.

There is a down side that I have heard nothing about and that is in addition to broken glass, how about when there is a change in the weather? As summer blends into fall and on, the rains come with a little snow and I don't enjoy cold feet. If you get used to running barefooted in slush will you feel normal running on bare smooth dry surfaces when the weather permits? I think you should try shoes first and for me, last, too.

In shoe discussions there is usually someone who reminds others of the Olympic Marathon that was won by a runner running barefooted. His name is Abebe Bikila from Ethiopia and he holds the record as the only winner of two

Summer Olympic Marathons and countless others. Perhaps it's the air in Ethiopia that makes him such an outstanding barefooted athlete. Good for him, but no thank you for me. During the week when I am not running, I use old running shoes and save the expensive conventional shoes for dress. Find a running store in your area and ask for shoe and general running advice. Tell them I sent you.

Lap 10 ~ When Your Breath Comes in Short Pants

After running for several years I read an article by the famous Dr. George Sheehan in which he suggests that most runners constrict abdominal muscles while inhaling. He suggests relaxing those abs while inhaling and contracting while exhaling. Try it. It makes a lot of sense but at first you have to concentrate on it to make it happen.

Deeper than normal breathing may bring in a little more air and therefore oxygen to your lungs and that brings hyperventilating to mind. All it means is more rapid and perhaps deeper breathing. It stands to reason that if a runner can circulate blood that is richer in oxygen he or she should be able to nourish all tissues of the body to advantage. I have tried several efforts that seem to help. One such for a fast race ending is to breathe twice as fast as you would normally starting a few hundred meters before the end of a race and right to the finish. It requires a little time to add oxygen to your blood stream so start hyperventilating well before the end.

A suggestion that has been helpful to me from time to time is to purse your lips while exhaling as if you were blowing out the candles on your grandchildren's (great grandchildren's) birthday cakes. That effort may force more oxygen out of the air and into your bloodstream.

Lap 11 ~ A Stitch in Time

In training, anything reasonable I read or heard about I tried during my three times a week hourly workouts. One runner suggested I run for endurance. To do it I would have to run for a distance, say three miles one day and add a mile the next workout. This was my high injury period at which I would forget the "take it easy" advice and I had one injury after another.

At races I would ask other runners if they had ever had the symptoms I was currently experiencing. Waiting for a race at Quinnipiac University, I mentioned one problem I had and I presume she was an instructor in physical culture asked me if I carried a wallet in a back pocket. I thought she was about to ask for a donation. I answered that I did and she said, "Take it out. You describe a condition called, in the literature, "Thick Wallet Disease." I changed pockets and after a couple of months the pain was gone.

Sprinting uphill one day, I knew I had a problem with a sudden pain in my left lower leg. That was unfortunate as I could not run in races. A swelling in my Achilles tendon of the left leg took almost six months to be able to run on and another two years for the swelling to be gone.

Another painful experience was in my right buttocks and that one brought me to our family doctor, Dr. Robert Gordon, who elected to have me examined with x-rays. He read part of the report to me. "You have osteoarthritis in and around both hips and up and down your back with two protruding intervertebral discs and my advice to you is to do whatever you want to do because that's what you will do anyway." I love Dr. Gordon, who is retired now.

Apparently it is due to the arthritis that I run bent forward and it seems there is nothing I can do about it. I mention that problem to exemplify that most anatomical problems should not prevent you from running. It seems to me that if I can do it, almost everyone should be able to do it.

I will never know if all those injuries were due to overtraining because of my age but I mention them as an example of the value of taking it easy and, when and if you have a problem, be advised that you too may be able to let nature help correct it but don't give up the ship for a few injuries. For the past five years I have had absolutely no problems that necessitate taking it easy. At this writing I am only 92 years old and as I age perhaps I'll change my mind.

Lap 12 ~ You May Shrink

Have you checked your weight lately? In high school I was a wrestler in the 155 pound class meaning that I had to remain under 158 pounds. Soon after college and after returning from the military in WWII, I weighed 189 pounds and a little more from time to time. At age 80 when I decided to run "to get in shape," I weighed 183 pounds and that was within the published acceptable range for one of my age and height.

With running and training, I soon began to wonder how much better I might run if I lost 10 pounds. After all, think of running with a 10-pound bag of flour on your back. It was not actually a diet to lose weight but I thought about my experiences in my veterinary practice. I had advised owners of overweight pets to reduce their pet's diet by 50 percent. A few would actually do it and return in a week to weigh their animals on our large platform scale. Most of the animals would not have lost an ounce and for some time I assumed someone was slipping the starving animals food perhaps under the table. It was not so. I found the animals had been eating over twice the amount necessary for the exercise they were getting.

I began to look at food differently than in the past. Looking at food I would think, "If I eat less I may be able to run better." That thinking and the exercise resulted in 170 pounds and it kept going down to 150 pounds where I have been for several years. Some runners my height and age weigh 140 pounds so that is my goal at this time.

Many race directors include special classes for heavy individuals and some call the class, "Clydesdales," consisting of remarkable athletes. Never have I seen a heavy senior runner in that class. Don't let that discourage you if you are one.

Lap 13 ~ Never Trust a Naked Runner

Basically the purpose of running attire is to cover parts of the human anatomy, and some of the extremes in accomplishing that are interesting to see. The costumes add to the upbeat atmosphere of the event. Starting with the shoes, perhaps the need is to cover the bare feet and, as I mentioned previously, there are those who wear no shoes but most have shoes with style in color and design that have only to do with attracting the runner to that brand and nothing to do with function. Some pants are loose and some are skin tight. Some are long and some short and of any and all colors. The shirts are in a category all of their own inscribed with political preference, commercial stuff, old racing accomplishments and some have strange quotations.

Have you ever wondered how you might feel dressed in running attire? Once you start you will experience a strange difference that is part of the running mystique. You are never too old to try.

When the temperature dips below about 50 degrees F. many runners start covering bodies with nylon "silks" before appropriate outer clothing. The silks serve a function as well as warmth. When a runner falls s/he is less apt to skin knees or elbows and I speak from experience.

My wife and I were dining at an annual Audubon dinner when I felt a hand on my shoulder and turning found

Melinda Struwas, a very attractive young woman runner and consistent trophy winner who said, "Doc Whitney, I thought it was you but I didn't recognize you with your clothes on."

With all the clothing originality there is one item worn with no special effects and that is the color of the socks. To try to address that observation I wear different colored socks. Hmmm.

It was 45 years ago I watched and timed my late wife folding my socks and neatly putting them in a dresser drawer. I figured that in 20 years of weekly folding my socks she would have spent over a month, 24 hours a day folding socks. I thought that was unacceptable and asked her to put them unfolded in a drawer and I would pick out a pair to wear. I have worn different colored socks since.*

* See Appendix 4, page 153

Lap 14 ~ Doin' What Comes Naturally

In answer as to what to do with your hands while running may be of curious interest and nothing more. I am told big time coaches of young competitive racers tell them to hold their hands as if holding a raw egg in each hand. The shells should not be cracked. I suggest doing what comes naturally. Never to be overlooked is what you wear on those hands while communing with nature. Wonderful light weight gloves that can hold a ton of water while running in the rain has to be a consideration. I tried mittens but they are too awkward. Your running store folks will help with proper gloves for any occasion.

What to do with the arms seems more important because establishing your own particular rhythm is discovered during your first jogging period. Some swing their arms until each hand is almost in their mouths. It seems to me that "it don't mean a thing if you ain't got that swing." I suggest you develop a swing of arms that seems most comfortable and you will discover the arm swing is an important part of smooth running.

Lap 15 ~ To Top It Off

Some would, given a choice, die rather than wear a hat. What you do about it is entirely a matter of choice but I enjoy shade from the sun so a visor seems appropriate. A sweatband helps keep the juices from running into eyes so a combination is my choice but the choice is a personal one. They can be costly or a bandana, twisted and knotted for your head size is an inexpensive sweatband solution. Dark glasses may be helpful.

Some running directors choose days for races that are so windy that just to keep a hat on your head is a major problem. In my climate some choose race days so close to zero temperature that ear coverings are a necessity. A hat can prevent frozen ears. So, let weather, personality, style and utility be your choice just as it is with your socks.

Lap 16 ~ Stopwatch Love-and-Hate Device

A stopwatch is truly a love/hate instrument. The cost can be so ridiculously low there is little reason to avoid them. You can love one when you have excelled at a given distance and the opposite when you are too slow. It is satisfying to find that after workouts your times improve and it is also pleasurable to leave the instrument home when you go for a gentle "conversation" mode run. In an organized run there is little advantage as your time is called out at the first mile and sometimes at every mile during the event. Organized running at a fun speed is next.

Lap 17 ~ Go to College

Older runners don't have to be as old as I am but if so, or if your balance is as unpredictable as mine is, you may prefer running on a running track. When I started, at 80 years of age, I ran on old tote roads on what was previously a water authority property purchased by our town of Orange. On hilly areas, rain would wash out ruts and leaves would fill in making a treacherous trail to maneuver. I fell 5 times on those runs, and on the last time I fell twice on the same day within 100 yards of each other.

We have several heavily traveled local vehicle roads in my town and many of the small roads are too narrow to feel safe running on. I decided to run on a track. Most high schools have tracks and the Yale University tracks were only a mile and a half from my house at the time. The University elders permit athletes of all stripes to use their perfectly maintained track at no charge when it is not in use by their athletes. If you are fortunate enough to have an institute of higher learning or a high school in your area, try them. For the University it is the best community outreach I can imagine.

At the Yale 400-meter outdoor track the inner of eight lanes is 400 meters. That means four times around the inner lane makes almost a mile. It's easy to keep track of the distances traveled and my stopwatch keeps me informed as to my progress. On the outside track Coach Dickerson calls the outer laps "bonus laps" when I run lane eight and then seven and so forth down to and including lane one. He calls that two miles but it has to be a bit over two. Then I start on lane four and run it and three, two and one to make a total of three-plus miles. Miles that are in excess of a 5k race. When I run those 12 laps during the week, I feel ready for a 5k race on the weekend.

Many universities and colleges have indoor running facilities available to the public at specified times during months of bad weather. I run on one provided by Smith College in Northampton, Mass. It is a 200-meter, six-lane oval with four tennis courts inside the laps. Yale's 200-meter inside facility is no longer available to the public. Indoor running is nothing short of a luxury with freezing rain, snow and sleet outside.

An important advantage of track running is that a runner does not have to look down at feet to prevent tripping over varied obstacles. Proper posture for running seems to be looking at the horizon and in an erect stance. Training on tote roads and even side roads necessitates looking for obstacles. The only obstacle on the tracks is you. Perhaps you should try track running. If you have a "rails to trails" * development near you, that seems to me to be an excellent solution.

When running on local roads it is always important to know that, statistically, every so many vehicles is operated

*See Lap 31, page 58

by someone who has no business driving because of drugs, the worse of which is alcohol. Some older drivers should be off the roads and some heavy-footed youngsters should be restrained, too. If you must run on auto traveled roads, dress to be obvious and with lights at night. Above all, please run toward oncoming traffic.

Lap 18 ~ Use Tact, Fathead

Training on a busy track presents problems, or does it? When a track was busy with runners in training, being age-slow I tried to get out of the way of everyone else since most everyone is faster than I am. Some were being timed by coaches. One day after a workout a coach who had seen me avoiding fast lanes of the track asked me to hear his advice. "When you are training on any track always remember age has precedence over all runners. Do not alter your program for any of the other runners."

Since then I do my workouts and let the younger runners avoid me and not the other way around. Of course when a track meet is going on, the word "TRACK" is shouted for any who are on the track during an event. It's like "FORE" in golf, in case you have heard of that "exercise" intensive hobby. A slogan on one running shirt reads, "No, I don't play golf. That's for older people."

Lap 19 ~ Run Like You Stole Something

An obvious result in aging seems to me to be the loss of "knee-lift." Older runners such as Ed Whitlock of Ontario, Canada, and Bill Tribou from Granby, CT, still have remarkable knee lift. I have tried workouts stressing knee lift and believe it is of more help in older runners' training than most workouts. The fact that running with exaggerated knee-lift is so damned difficult may be a tip that I need more of it. If you are a new older runner there is little doubt in my mind that you will improve your general ability by working on it. After a warm-up, run one straight way of a track with knees rising high until it seems difficult and coast perhaps around the curve of the track and repeat it. If you do that exercise many times, I can practically guarantee you will feel it at least the following morning when you try to get out of bed. Of course, such fatigue indicates a worthwhile workout.

As you stride out running, it seems natural that you will wonder about the length of your stride. I wonder how much time might be improved by taking a half inch longer stride in say a mile run. I find it more tiring to force a longer stride than seems most comfortable and I doubt the effort is worth it, but each of us marches to our own drummer. Here again, each of us must determine the best stride, knee-lift and rapidity of stride for ourselves.

Here seems to me to be an impossible situation. You

have a schedule of exercise you have agreed with yourself to stick to when one day you believe as your brain dictates that you cannot jog that scheduled time because your legs are too stiff or tired or you are just not up to it. Let's say the exercise you are up to is 100 paces of walking and the same of jogging. You go out and start with the walking and after the walking you automatically start the jogging effortlessly and enjoyably. You are doing what your brain has told you that you cannot do.

In that situation your brain has misinformed you and your body contradicts the message from it. How is that possible? It would seem that there must be something wrong with your brain chemistry. It isn't a problem, it's normal for everyone, it seems to me. It is worth knowing that at times we should overlook the message from our brains and allow our bodies to tell us if a negative message was valid.

Lap 20 ~ Who Are You?

Let me attempt to predict who is taking the time to read this document. You are interested in maintaining reasonably good health or improving your not-so-good health. You have been subjected to so many references of the importance of exercise you wonder what this author thinks he has as an answer. If you are a man or woman still able to do normal housework, you are a potential runner. If you are a man or a woman who can still mow the lawn or do a little yard work you are a potential runner. If you can walk to the bus or put the trash out or if you could bowl again or if you can still walk to the local watering hole you are a potential runner. If you have to climb a staircase off and on and probably if you are curious as to why your friends would read this, you may be the first one on your block to actually dig out those old sneakers and try it yourself.

Even if you have minor discomfort in joints and they tell you that your joint cartilage is wearing out or even if they say your bones are rubbing together, you could be amazed to find that by exercise alone you may start to regenerate rather than the degenerating that faces you in the future with lack of exercise. From personal experience I can tell you that from over exerting rather than taking it easy, I have improved at least half a dozen injuries in my legs. I found that by continuing running, the corrective ability of my body responded with complete recovery in each case. A couple of those injuries took six months of very slow running.

Once you take up the sport you will have many choices of what you would like to be called. We are called senior runners or mature runners or elders or oldsters or old timers or some call us "third act" runners. Of course we are master runners to some and old fogies to others. I've seen the words gold, silver and platinum used, too. There comes a problem in who calls us what. More important to me is what you call yourself. Often such a state of existence is set at age 65. What does matter is the sound of the remark. If it's disparaging, someone is uninformed.

It's entirely possible and may be probable that the winner in an older age group registered a time that was a winning record time for his or her age group and perhaps for the race. That would not be known ever unless a great deal of work was done in establishing worldwide times for all age groups. I predict one day it will happen. You may have a grandson who could work up a computer program to enable a race director to come up with not only the age group winners but the real winners of each race. What an incentive for all age runners who feel like it to compete.

I will expound more on this later.

Lap 21 ~ To Push Your Car Over

Before a running event or when a group of runners gather before a workout it is interesting to watch many trying to push trees, buildings, fences and even their cars over. Some are on their backs pulling first one leg and then the other right out of their hip sockets. Some of those calisthenics last over half an hour and many swear by them.

Watch some of them and try them yourself. I've done just that and find that I think I should save all the energy I can muster for the event, be it practice or a race. My policy is to emulate my coach, Chris, who half an hour before a race runs at quite a pace for ten minutes and then takes it easy until race time. Personally I take a 10-minute easy jog half an hour before a race. It seems to me that if you have been working out regularly, you are ready for a race anytime without the pre-race workouts.

High school and college coaches often put their charges through half an hour of miscellaneous exercises before permitting them to engage in serious exercise. Many elders should try stretching to perhaps loosen stiff joints to good advantage and I have been so advised by coaches repeatedly. You be the judge.

Lap 22 ~ Walk and Run

Stop by a bookstore and note the number of books devoted to aspiring runners written by proven runners and coaches. There are dozens if not hundreds of them. Many have adventure themes and most are written to attempt to convince readers that a given great reached his or her pinnacle by some system of training experiences that he or she apparently thinks would be best for you.

The very fact that there are so many books and so many varied suggestions should tell us something. With all the information available it still comes to mind, does much of it relate to individual *older* runners? I don't think science has addressed that question and I have a good deal of trust in science as well as in my coaches.

I noticed one runner who is of an age almost reaching maturity (about 50, I would think), who in many races walked for a hundred paces or so and then broke into a run. Using that system I would pass him while he walked and he would pass me when he ran. He would invariably beat me at the end. I asked him about his system and he explained that a year before he had had a triple heart bypass surgery and was getting into shape by running.

I asked my coach, Chuck, and he assured me that system was not as productive as steady running to the end. Recently, having decided on a speed workout, I tried jogging the loops of the track and running "hard" for the straight-aways. It seemed to me that I ran a faster 5k during that training period and I am tempted to try it in an official race. It is possible that the experience of Coach Chuck with high school youngsters is, in this case, not applicable to we oldsters.

I realized I was repeating my earlier experience when starting when I would walk a hundred paces and run a hundred. This time I would jog a hundred and run a fast hundred. Hmmm. As I have said all along that beauty is in the eye of the beholder when the beholder is a runner.

Lap 23 ~ An Idea Who's Time Has Come

At this point all readers recognize that this book is accepting the awesome challenge of attempting to change long established habits of sedentary elders. Perhaps that is an impossibility but perhaps the advantages are well enough delineated to accomplish enough encouragement to get a few gutsy individuals, both men and women, to try the suggestions. If so, others will follow.

It has been said that an idea whose time has come is more powerful than any army. The evidence of better health and longer life for elders is so convincing that the idea of seniors jogging and running may be one of the great ideas whose time has come in spite of the negativism so rampant in society.

With a small number of individuals having discovered the validity of the idea by being personally involved with jogging and running the stage may be set for a mass acceptance for even a majority of non-runners.

Lap 24 ~ Grandma Running?

You should anticipate problems on the horizon before they seem insurmountable. One such may happen when the middle-aged mother brings the copy of this book home and grandma, age 80, who is living with the family picks it up and quietly reads it and makes some plans for herself. What will both the mother and father and the two high-school-age children have to say about grandma going out and running around the neighborhood? She can't do that. What will the neighbors say? Forget what the neighbors will say, Grandma may say, "never mind the neighbors I want to try that crazy veterinarian's prescription for growing old more gracefully."

I love you, Grandma. I'll run with you anytime.

And then the new elderly couple to the neighborhood who on finishing the book decides to at least try the insurance policy and is seen three times a week walking and suddenly jogging for a few paces at first and in a month are jogging 100 paces between similar numbers of walking paces. Should something be done about them?

However, if a careful analysis is made, it will be found that the old folks who try this adventure will tell the neighbors, politely, to join them or to go to… read the book.

Let it now be known that this book has the possibility of becoming a new Bible for older seniors. Will you be included?

Lap 25 ~ Publications

Among the mountains of books on the subject of running, there are few books for older runners and I have found only one book written by an older runner who started as an old man and that is, *Come Jog With Me*. As far as magazines for runners, you may enjoy reading of exploits of many great athletes but other than admiration and wonderment if you started in your younger years and might be among the greats today, there is little to benefit the likes of us. Out of the thousands of those like us, I predict there will be a limited number to attempt to excel in speed for our ages and therefore will not be newsworthy.

Different strokes for different folks are applicable here. Most new runners should do it for no other reason than it is pleasant and, oh, so invigorating. A very few may find pleasure in trying to excel and that's great if your kicks come from more than competition with yourself.

As far as magazines are concerned, I enjoy those for all ages of us and some that are regional. There is one published by the USATF (United States Track and Field)* that zeros in on the likes of us. It covers field as well as track but it emphasizes running of older athletes. For members it publishes the names of those who mature into an older age group as each reaches their new birthday designation. That one is *The Masters News*.* They also have a New England all-

*See Appendix 9, Page 165

age publication. So far there is no magazine specifically for new older runners like us but with my prediction of masses of older runners soon to be involved, someone will establish an over 65 age running magazine for us and I urge you to subscribe when that egg hatches. We can count on more publications with the constant expansion of numbers of runners of all ages.

Lap 26 ~ The Fair Sex

Concerning women runners, I hope one day soon an older woman will write a book of running for older non-running women. Although this book is for all sexes I feel presumptuous in attempting to cover areas of the sport from the female vantage point. I ask women runners and non-runners to be kind to me and know I appreciate my shortcomings in this area.

A lot of water has gone over the dam since women started running in numbers. Before I started to run 10 years ago, I observed women running on roads with a gait not quite running and not quite fast walking. It was sort of a shuffle gait almost like a fast duck's gait. A coach would shudder and lecture about "knee lift" among other things to such an athlete. Recently while working out, a woman appeared on the Yale track with a lap of jogging after which she "took off" and while I ran for eight laps she must have done 18. She had a fantastic stride with two shades of lavender for a costume and her long hair dancing with each stride. It was a memorable sight.

These days it is not a rarity for a woman to run races faster than the fastest male. In long races such as a hundred miles, women often excel. I wonder why. It was a woman runner who suggested a slogan for one of my running shirts, "MOTHER TOLD ME NEVER TO ASSOCIATE WITH

FAST WOMEN."

It comes to mind that rarely do I see a woman runner in her seventies. I haven't any idea why there are not more female vintage runners. In Connecticut, Monica Roach and Patty Carton happen to be exceptions and even after having been side swiped by a car, after a convalescent period, Monica is back running at over 70 years of age. Alas, I see all too few male runners at or over 70 years of age. Both women and men non-runners do not realize their latent ability to be able to run even starting at 80 as I have done. It just may be that senior women runners are anatomically better suited than males of the same age for distant running and perhaps for field events, too. Maybe 10 years or so from now, I'll know if you start giving me competition.

Lap 27 ~ Workouts and Persistence

As far as ideas presented here are concerned, you may rest assured that many were lifted from other runners. If ideas work for you use them and discard the others. If you are interested in improving (who isn't?) that means workouts or training. In my mind there may be problems in training with programs used for younger runners that may not apply to the likes of us. I read many running magazines but few books with so few older runners writing about the sport.

Without older runners publishing their ideas it seems to me we must improvise. A series of workouts that seem to work for me may not be appropriate for you but may give you some ideas. For many months I practiced on a "rails to trails" * project in a neighboring town. That worked out well for me as there are no motorized vehicles permitted and the miles are marked on the blacktop.

Early on, when I could jog two miles without stopping, the schedule consisted of running out from my parked car for a mile and then back. After resting a day or two, I would increase the distance by half a mile with each workout. In two months a 5k (3.1 miles) distance was no problem. After my early races I would rest two days and repeat the 5k on the rails-to-trails trail. Coach Dickerson then advised some speed workouts and on the Yale 200-meter track, I was told to warm up by a couple of slow

*See Lap 31, page 58

jogs around the track, to rest and then to try to sprint around lane eight and rest for about two minutes and repeat the effort on lane seven. Repeat it for all eight lanes and rest for two days.

The morning after the first speed workout, my wife asked why I was grunting as I tried to extricate myself from the bed clothes.

It was about a year after starting organized racing that, at age 81, I finally ran in a 5k race in just under 30 minutes. It has never happened again. Now at age 90, my objective is to run every 5k in under 50 minutes. Be assured, if I had not kept up the exercise my ability would be far less than it is today.

As I repeat several times, it is critical to keep a training schedule and not fail it. Of course whatever works for you, stick to it. Occasionally I get out to the track and decide I just don't feel like running today. Then I start to warm up and the urge to "JUST DO IT!" takes over and I smile and finish the scheduled workout. Some days I decide to run at a slower pace than usual. One with which I can sing or have a conversation with myself. I recite Kipling's "Gunga Din" or "The Wreck of the Hesperus" out loud smiling all the way. Try your own poetry and you may like it but it's the more strenuous workouts that really slow the age-related slowing down.

On returning from a workout or race, don't hesitate to relax and sleep a little. I find my naps after workouts are a rapid deep sleep.

A habit pattern develops so that if I vacation from exercise I still experience deep sleep at nap or bedtime.

If you become active, try as I have to stay awake in bed to enjoy your newfound improvement in physical condition. I discovered that deep sleep comes in spite of trying to stay awake. This is an important additional plus for running for the fun of it.

Lap 28 ~ Can Runners Smile?

Once I sent a letter to the editor of my daily paper in which I wondered why members of a symphony orchestra never seemed to appear happy even when and after playing magnificent music. All except Itzhak Perlman who does smile after playing a difficult section. After that letter was published I found out that by letters of objection to mine when playing seriously, all musicians are so dedicated to excellence they do not smile. Before I started to run I thought the same about runners and I am sure every runner is asked the question from time to time. "Why don't you ever see runners smiling?"

I don't run on the roads in training in busy Connecticut. But while in Vermont off and on I do run the roads and I smile and wave to every oncoming vehicle and the drivers in better than nine out of 10 vehicles return my wave and I suspect many smile back. Think about it, do you see bowlers smiling while throwing the ball? Soccer players in the midst of the contest? Or even choirs in church if you attend church? Or bocce, curling or ping pong?

Most runners are serious about running well, as are other sports people while competing in their sports. After most sporting events there is plenty of laughter and smiles. With the sport of running, everybody is welcome to enjoy race gatherings that will prove the point. Even non-runners are usually welcome to join in the post-race festivities and refreshments.

Come to think of it, Andre Rieu's musicians do smile some while playing, excepting the horn players.

Lap 29 A Mystique

An example of the warmth found at races was a race that fell on my birthday in 2005. I pre-registered and race director Schiavonne noticed the coincidence and spread the word. Someone actually went to NYC and had shirts printed with "Happy Birthday, Doc George" and also with some of my slogans. At the race I was well wished by one after another runner. I noticed most had different colored socks on. During the race a mass of friends and well wishers ran behind me and let the record show how many I beat time wise. Then the frosting on the birthday cake was a huge cake with a copy of me running in color on the frosting. Really, runners are a fantastically warm group of people. People in all walks of life and no one is considered on the basis of color or station or occupation but environmentalists are always out in force when conversation touches on it.

When you try to get involved with racing, the friends you will make will delight you. The anticipation of upcoming races and training periods add an extra flavor to life that is serendipitous. Each race has a life of its own and at the conclusion may be a highlight of the year. Work for it and you will revel in your results.

For your first race and several thereafter, be advised to seek out the director and tell him or her I suggested that you join in. Explain that you are new to the sport. After the race you will be singled out as a new member of our sport.

Lap 30 ~ Cramps

Here is a subject that may cause you to question everything else written in this book. It's about cramps. The question of the cause of cramps is an interesting one. Science can put a man on the moon but cannot find the explanation of common conditions such as hiccups, cramps and sneezing. In our New Haven newspaper a Peter Gott, MD, publishes what often seems like "way out" suggestions for home remedies. Over the past several years he has reported that many readers have found a method of either preventing cramps or at least minimizing them. When first mentioned it was claimed that by putting a cake of soap under the bottom bed sheet, cramps would be a thing of the past.

Having had my share of cramps my thoughtful wife put a cake of soap under the sheet in our bed against my "better judgment." After six months or so she discontinued the soap as a joke. One night after both a strenuous running workout and then hauling logs for several hours, I had the most painful cramps I had ever had. I paced the floor and wondered about the soap and about anything that might alleviate the pain. In desperation I unwrapped a new bar of soap and inhaled it deeply. In about 10 minutes the cramps had subsided 100 percent. Since that time I keep a small bar of soap in my pajama pocket and have had few and light cramps if any.

Most home remedies are soon forgotten usually because

there is no scientific truth to be had in effectiveness and co-incidence has to be included in explanations. We do know inhaling substances can have a profound effect on all mammals. Examples are ether and other gas anesthetics. Then we have aphrodisiacs such as pheromones and perfume. Then there is camphor for fainting and cannabis for fun and medical purposes. Why not soap for cramps?

One day on an expedition to Mount Monadnock in New Hampshire to locate the best trail to attempt to climb that mountain, I suddenly decided to climb the White Arrow Trail without notifying my "keeper" daughter, Lee. The attempt was fun but also a disaster in that although I ascended to well above the tree line I elected to descend with the little energy I had left before I reached the top. My 91-year-old legs all but gave out. Thinking gravity would be helpful, I slowly picked my way down to almost the end when a State Park Ranger appeared to help me the rest of the way. My legs were so tired and with a cramp in my driving right leg I wondered if I could manage the 40-mile drive. Once home I stretched out on my bed ready to pass out in a deep sleep when I wondered about cramps. It was a struggle to my feet and some deep inhaling of a bar of soap before sleep that may have completely prevented cramps.

As far as I am concerned, the evidence indicates that the inhaling of soap fumes is effective in both preventing and retarding cramps and until there is other evidence I stand convinced.

As a scientist I can only repeat what others have claimed about results even if the mechanism is unknown. It seems to me that it works for me and, for you, you can try it to find out if it helps. Amen.

Also it should be mentioned that quinine is helpful. Ask an M.D. about that.

Lap 31 ~ Rails to Trails

A few more words about "rails to trails" mentioned previously. It is not only on old abandoned train tracks but on roadways where draft animals pulled barges along canals as well as old roads superseded by newer highways that trails are being developed. On such trails there is no motorized equipment to interfere with biking, hiking, strolling or even running. Slowly many of those lanes are being linked so that in the near future in my state of Connecticut a runner will be able to run through four towns and a city with only a couple of highway crossings consisting of 25 miles or more.

Although the rails to trails I used to run on traverse heavily commercial areas, I have seen lots of wildlife even a coyote and deer many times, rabbits and the occasional turtle heading out to lay her eggs. In hot weather with the trees meeting overhead it's a few degrees cooler and, oh, so pleasant.

Such a development in your area is well worth encouraging and supporting.

Lap 32 ~ Pick It Up a Little

Here are a few suggestions that seem helpful to me that I stumbled on over my months of running. In an early race I started to pass an elderly woman going up a hill who, I found out later, was 69 years old who spoke up and said, "Sonny, when running up hills you should take shorter strides." When I glanced at her face, she looked at me and seemed surprised and said, "Whoops!" Whatever that means. It was a common sense remark I have appreciated ever since. Try short strides up hills.

While being coached for an attempt at a run at Reggie Lewis Stadium in Boston about two thirds of the way around the track Coach Dickerson said, "Pick it up a little, Doc." And ever since in most races if I feel a bit strained or tired that voice returns and instead of slowing I smile and "pick it up." Incidentally I won silver for that race in Boston.

One of the excellent runners I see regularly complained of a shoelace coming untied during one race. He was fuming. It was a race in which we had chips for timing and perhaps the chip contributed. In training I had the same problem and decided to find a solution. The great runner Bill Rogers tells us he always double ties his laces. When I finish a race I have to admit I have almost too little energy to fight untying my double tied laces and decided to investigate finding a small clip to fasten to the knot. Then while mentioning the problem to my friend, Mike Buchina, a persistent 5k runner and friend, he gave me the tip I have used ever since with 100 percent success. By taking the inside loop of the tied lace and tucking it under one of the cross laces toward the toe of my shoe, the problem has been solved. Even with a timing chip laced in. I have decided I'm never too old to learn. How about you?

Lap 33 ~ The Reggie Lewis Stadium

My first running season completed, I turned my efforts to training. It was great fun and onlookers were lavish with their praise of my ability. Of course, I was skeptical about many friends complimenting me. Some insisted that if I were to go to an important Masters Meet in Boston in March they would guarantee I would win at least one medal. I convinced myself to try it.

It was an exciting event for me with my daughter, Carolyn, and her husband, John, coming from New York and coach-son Chuck from northern Maine, as well as my bride, Dorothy, as a cheering section. In retrospect I wonder if they wondered if at my age I might collapse on the track and be present for the service.

Even for non-runners a track meet at the famous Reggie Lewis Stadium is an exciting affair. That event is worth the trip just to watch the action. I saw some humor in the ending of the 1500-meter race when another runner passed me as we approached the finish. I knew only one of us would win the second place award and picked up my pace and as I gained the 3,000 spectators in the stands rose shouting and cheering us on. Two old age-slow bastards trying to outdo each other seemed funny to me. I beat him by half a step. And, yes, I did win not one but three medals.

Don't you wonder about how many untried senior runners

could do it and do it better than I? I do. You may be one.

There are several methods of timing runners at races. With few runners, as one recently here in Brattleboro, Vermont, a stopwatch is started at the start. At the end, the time is called out as each runner crosses the finish line.

With larger races of several hundred runners and up, the timing is done electronically with a time clock started when the starting gun or foghorn goes off, and out on the course another clock at mile one informs runners of their times for the first mile and at the conclusion by the starting clock.

With the age of electronics in some races, each runner has a chip attached to one shoelace. The time is recorded electronically at the finish line.

Lap 34 ~ A Running Partner?

Of course, the ideal may be to have a spouse for a running mate but that is not always possible. A friend of similar age and ability is a pleasure to run with in training or in a scheduled race. Oh, to find a senior of like mind and age and ability in one area may be impossible. Clubs feature training sessions for all.

Do not let the unavailability of someone like you discourage you from getting in shape to run a little. From experience you may find it an advantage to run alone. Alone you can change a planned workout at will, try an extra lap or idea not planned with someone else.

If competition is sought after, you may find the only competition is with your own past times for an event. There is, however, more and more competition in the over-70 year groups. With two non-runners starting to run together with my program, you have an excellent situation and if all the residents of the "Solace for all Retirement rest home" start together, Nova or National Geographic is apt to film you for posterity.

Lap 35 ~ A Family Sport

Running is a family sport in many families. My oldest daughter, Carolyn Sabol, decided if her father could do it, so could she. With her husband, John, she arrived to run in a 5k race with me. I did beat her in that race but, unbeknown to us, her husband ran and beat us both handily.

At one race an attractive young-looking woman struck up a conversation to inform me that her college-age daughters were runners and she had decided if I could run at 80 years of age, she should be able to, too. Now the three of them run regularly together. Such conversations are constant and welcome.

My two grandsons seem to have made the same observations and have become runners. One, Leon, is "top of the line." It is great to see children grow up to exceed both parents in their running or any other ability. It is also great to see older non-runners develop to outdo their children, until their grandchildren beat them.

It seems to me that this competitive sport is a wonderful sport for family togetherness, as well as an extra childhood experience about which any child can have bragging rights as well as good health. And there are bragging rights of parents and grandparents and I am a great-grandparent. On another level we older runners, no matter how slow, have bragging rights but more importantly know we are doing something worthy of bragging about.

Lap 36 ~ About Exercise

About exercise. It has always seemed to me that to exercise means to sweat. I know the experts say that we burn the same number of calories if running for a given distance as if we walk the same distance. Let's grant that fact although it is questionable to me. When exercise results in excess sweating, there has been a great deal more accomplished than so called "exercise" with no excess sweating. More about this later.

We know that urine and sweat are almost identical in makeup. We also know when the kidneys are not functioning properly, sweating helps remove waste materials from the blood. So, sweating to take the load off the kidney function may be helpful. Walking must be better than nothing but to equate it with running is to lose sight of reality. We all do sweat even in frigid weather but evaporation dissipates it.

Doing all sorts of calisthenics and motions with arms and legs should not be confused with physical exercising although a huge industry has sprung up that confuses social activities with real physical exercise.

In discussing exercise with myself I have come to some strange conclusions to the question, "What is enough?" I have answered by suggesting TIE or making your own decisions as when to TIE. But the answer to what is too much leads to other questions. In my early training I insisted in overdoing that resulted in a string of injuries with a string of recoveries. In a race in Trumbull, Conn., I started my race-ending sprint too early and one step before the finish line collapsed. The medics helped me to my shaky legs and to their rescue vehicle. In two or three minutes, I arose and left the van to jog into the race headquarters. Aftereffects? There were none.

Reading about a super-human effort, Laurie Andrews of Jackson Hole, Wyoming, ran in a Super Marathon of 150 miles. In that race the runners sleep six hours and run on. At about 120 miles she could hold little in her stomach and she hid behind brush to eat and promptly lose the food she had eaten. She wondered if she were damaging herself but continued to the end. She not only finished but with her 36 hours and 22 minutes, she was the fastest of any American woman with no aftereffects.

It seems to me that if you are in shape for the exercise of running, it is impossible to overdo. You have seen, on television, Olympic distance skiers collapse at the end of a race and even before the end with no ill effects. If anatomically unprepared for an activity, anyone can over do and with pre-existing medical problems, that is another matter.

If you love life with good health, a proven excellent exercise is running. On one of the running shirts I have, "If You Ain't Sweatin' It, You Ain't Gettin' It."

I talked with one runner who had a dry T-shirt after a 5k race in 80-degree weather and asked how come. He informed me that he does not sweat. So I guess I should not paint every runner with the same paint brush although for most the above holds.

I asked an old friend why he sits around all day? He said, "I believe in conservation and I'm conserving energy." Another excuse. Have you ever wondered why you have the hardware to be able to do what so many can and do like running? Our ancestors must have had to run from danger or perhaps run to catch up with food for the table. Like immunity we all have inherited remarkable anatomical accoutrements. On the other side of the coin, those ancestors who could not run fast enough are not in your or my pedigrees for good reason. On one of my running shirts I have, "RUN LIKE YOU STOLE SOMETHING."

It is interesting that the most common dream for all strains of humans is being chased. With our ability to run distances, could being able to run distances have saved our early human ancestors by running from pursuing danger?

Speaking of sweating reminds me that high on any diet list is the suggestion that adult humans should drink 6-8 glasses of water daily. With running advice the word, "hydration" is important because the loss of excess water and salt can be disastrous. Even for non-runners the water advice is important as the water is absorbed and circulates with the blood to be detoxified as it passes through detoxifying organs and before being passed off as sweat and urine. Obviously jogging or running adds to the amount of junk removal from the act of exercise and the resulting better health.

Lap 37 ~ Use It or Lose It

I think some older people would think because they are aging, say 65 years old, they could not run because of not having used it. Let's clear the air here, I am not talking about sex although that too is probably improved (it was in my case) with real exercise. In my case if that idiom, "Use It or Lose It," were valid at 80 I would not have run in that first race. The idiom older people who do not exercise might well put on their shirts is, "I CHOSE TO LOSE IT." That sounds shameful to me.

That does lead to another consideration so far untouched in this book that has had volumes written about it. That is the plight of so many of the older non-running generations in society. On the surface it appears that the majority of ageing people are striving to reach a point of doing nothing. That has to be, next to painful health problems, the ultimate tragedy in the final years of living. So here I am presenting a partial solution to boredom at a ridiculously low cost for everyone to embrace.

Nature does demand an end to all living things and crudely put, those who are too far gone cannot live to enjoy the art of running. So, many have convinced themselves against better judgment that they are in the final group when it "ain't necessarily so." For all potential runners, including those who know running is not for them, there is one carrot not emphasized that should be mentioned and that comes to me as the Leonardo De Vinci consideration. When that master sculptor completed his statues it was obvious he appreciated the stark nude anatomy of the human body. So the opportunity for runners of all sexes to admire the anatomical features of other humans is an unmentioned reason to enjoy the sport even with all the coverings.

There may be another reason for running even more compelling than others mentioned if you are a matriarch or patriarch of a family of sedentary offspring, and that is to take up the sport of running to set an example for those children, grandchildren and even great-grandchildren to emulate. Or even as an example by which to shame everybody under your age over your exploits to come run with YOU. We all know such families of couch potatoes and in that case you could be a lifesaver.

When you do try it, you may find a good slogan is, "ENJOY YOURSELF. THIS IS NO DRESS REHEARSAL." I'll look for you at a 5k race in a year or so.

Lap 38 ~ Running Thoughts

After jogging and running for a few years I found myself wondering what others think about while running. To find out I conducted a period of asking fellow exercisers what they thought. There were no surprises, as some couldn't recall what they thought about. One said he looks at any landmark ahead and runs to it and looks for another. One said he thought about a good-looking female he had been talking to before the race named Ilse. Several mentioned stride and speed and condition for the run. One said he saw Monica, age 71, ahead and picked up his pace. The only consistency was variety.

As far as my thoughts while running are concerned, mine too are a variety among which are two that are quite consistently present. About how I'm doing at the moment with my diet to lose weight. The thought is that by losing a few pounds I may be able to run with more ease. Incidentally I am down to 139.5 after a 5k training run. That has been my objective for a month – losing 10 pounds and I may keep going for 130 to test the waters. I also quite regularly think of my theories about our bodies requiring the elimination of toxic substances and I think about ridding my system of normal and abnormal waste material. The normal wastes are from normal food and water metabolism and the abnormal wastes are from food additives or indigestible foods and even medications. You will find more about this later on in the reading but I visualize a cup of toxic stuff being poured down a drain just by the running activity. Then I may think about the organs of my body involved. In any event, for me the thoughts are interesting and satisfying.

A question often asked of runners is, "Isn't running boring?" As compared with the extent of the boredom of many senior lives who just sit around, running is doing something constructive with time and considering the pre-jogging and the post-jogging activities, it is far from boring in addition to which the feeling of better health is an additional reward in itself.

Lap 39 ~ Singing in the Rain

I asked my coach son who is a professional grade wild bird enthusiast when the best time for finding birds to identify was and he replied, "When it's raining or not." The question comes to mind, when is the best time to run? For me the answer is the same as for birding. There are those who wonder at runners running in the rain. It is a given that race organizers sometimes cannot control the weather so those runners who have trained with that in mind are ready for most any weather. It was in one race during a period of high winds and driving sheets of rain that problems developed for me. Of the 300 to 400 runners expected, there were only about 55 who actually took to the road when that storm was at its peak. The first problem was that there were absolutely no runners over 60 years of age other than I at 87. So it was early on in the race that everybody had long since disappeared from my sight. The rain had washed all signs of the race away and so at a critical intersection, I turned the wrong way. It was along a road at the edge of Long Island Sound and in spite of my laughing about running in such weather when the rain was so thick, it even prevented an appreciation of the beauty of the scene. My laughing was short lived when the road ended in a cul-de-sac. I back tracked with no idea where in the City of Milford, Conn., I was.

My second problem besides being lost was that it was a

race being timed and would go down on my record. Fortunately there were also walkers at that race and I spotted both of them at the end of a long, straight street. They told me the general direction and I somehow ended up at the school where we had started. Strangely, my 40-minute time was not that bad. The second problem was that being so slow, would the food be gone? There was no problem with food at that race and all 55 of us were urged to take food to distribute to the needy.

Lap 40 ~ To Jog or Run

It is usually the well-endowed, well-trained runners who complain about runners who come to an organized race and rather than racing are jogging. With older runners, our slow times may place all of us in the jogging category even when we are giving the race our ultimate effort. For us to have some 50-year-old, slow-jogging youngsters we sometimes beat in a race adds a little incentive. I would think the numbers would be immaterial to the good young runners. If there are 100 or so joggers, they add numbers so the better racers can brag that they have placed over 400 others rather than 300 without commenting on the number of joggers in the race.

In each age group every runner has friends or acquaintances who become competitors in every race once the gun goes off. I believe there are few runners who permit their speed to be very far under their capable times.

With more and more physicians encouraging patients to run for all sorts of reasons, many slower runners are obeying doctor's orders. Many non-runners find their blood pressure decreases five or more points after a few months of running and many mention slower resting pulse rates.

Lap 41 ~ Guinea Pigs

A friend of mine whom I have never met and I have never even communicated with has become a friend because of medical research he reported in November 2009. His name is Dr. James Fries and he has headed a study group, observing 538 older runners for 20 years and a similar group of non-runners.

I will list some of the advantages Dr. Fries identified in runners over non-runners that are similar to what happened to me after starting at 80 years of age. Some of the statements may sound familiar if you have read much of *Come Jog with Me*.

1. The running exercise mentioned in his study extends active life.

2. Nineteen years after the beginning of the study, 34 percent of the non-runners had died and 15 percent of the runners.

3. The onset of disabilities came earlier in non-runners.

4. Some disabilities in runners came 16 years later than in non-runners.

5. Part of the reason for better health may have been eating habits and less weight.

Dr. Fries is 69 years old, a runner and is an outdoor person and the only person I know who has actually run a small lap around the North Pole. He is an emeritus professor associated with Stanford University in California. Eureka!

Lap 42 ~ Hill Running

From my readings, most runners of any age are uncomfortable with hill training or hill running. Just tackle hills head on. Find a hill with a rather steep grade at least 100 paces long and decide to love that particular hill. Then at least once every two weeks or less, attack it for about an hour.

Use your stopwatch and take an easy jog for the first 100 paces. Walk down and do it again but try to cover the distance in a shorter time. Keep that exercise up for the best part of an hour with your fastest times toward the end. I usually increase my speed gradually with each trip until I can no longer beat any of my previous times. For me, a couple of days after such a workout my legs feel great and I think it improves my speed. Try it. You may like it and appreciate it when confronted by a hill in an organized race.

It is comforting to know what to expect in hills in a new race. Many races have attractive descriptions like the daffodil race in Meridan, CT. I had not inquired about hills until just before the start. It was the lure of half a million daffodils in full bloom that enticed me as I am fond of beauty. After seeing those flowers in such profusion, I decided hills didn't matter until the course headed out of Daffodil Park and toward a mountain. I decided I was proud of myself in ascending that grade only to run 50 paces or so level to an extension of the first elevation and up an even steeper second one. Then, being almost at the end of my rope, we circled back down both slopes.

On the other hand, the Cow Bell 5k in East Haddam, CT, is special for older runners. I asked about the course, "Is it pancake flat?" In answer "No. It's up the mountain." Then showing my reaction, it was added, "Up the mountain by bus and down the 5k to almost the finish all downhill." My time was the year's best in that one.

Lap 43 ~ Cut and Run Bursts

Another training workout on a college or high school track consists of an easy run around lap eight and then cutting to lap seven and running the straightaway almost as fast as possible and, for me, that's 100 paces followed by a slow run around the curve to the next straightaway and another sprint and, at the lane seven to six, I call out "cut" and run at the next straightaway and keep that up until I have traveled 5k. That's 12 laps of an eight-lap running track and that means 24 sprints. Of course, if you're training on another surface instead of laps by alternating paces of 100 fast and slow, you have the same workout. In my case when I've used that system, my times in timed races have improved.

It just may be that the system is productive for older runners and not so for younger athletes. You may find it's not for you but again you be the judge. I think it's worth trying.

My friend Bill Tribou was one of the seven best milers in our country when in his young prime and has persisted, winning age groups constantly. He is in his 90's now and still setting age group records. He tells me he has had to walk for parts of every race for the last six months and is still setting age group records. So if you cannot run for a full 5k, know you are in good company.

Lap 44 ~ Research Anyone?

Wouldn't it be comforting for you if you knew your doctor was aware of some of the stuff you eliminate while running that might harm you if you were a non-runner? Today with the equipment in medical labs, they have machines that a few years ago could tell bad stuff if it was a millionth part in the sample and be glad that today the biochemist can tell if stuff is a billionth to one in a sample.

So here is a suggestion for your favorite research group. Have them contact race directors in your area to announce that at a given race, urine samples will be requested from before and after the race to help determine why runners are healthier than non-runners and samples will be requested from non-running others in attendance as control research animals.

Where I used to hang my hat, the Connecticut Agricultural Experiment Station has that sophisticated equipment and the scientists could do that study. Taking it a step further blood samples could be requested for further studies but the urine tests could be accomplished with less fuss in sampling.

Sometimes it takes a little prodding to get some important action moving. One person can make a difference and you may be that one person to get some action. You might organize such a project and in so doing revel in a scientific adventure.

The results of such a project could be to help convince non-runners to awaken to the fact that they, young or old, should run for the health of it.

For running to be such a constant and pronounced trait it must have been developed early on after leaving the jungle and before we spread all over this earth. Then comes the question of, if it is such a profoundly ancient gift, could other changes either good or bad be accompanied by that inherited trait of running? Could the brain chemistry be affected by the constant striking of each foot to the ground with each stride in running? If so, could running have an influence on our immune system that non-runners cannot enjoy?

Could brain chemistry have an effect on our having less Alzheimer's than non-runners? Less hardening of the arteries, atherosclerosis and the resulting strokes and heart problems? Shouldn't running be checked out before gene studies are undertaken as a preventive of such as Parkinson's? MS? MD? ALS? And Alzheimer's that my mother had the last three or four years before her death? I think so. It is my hope that this book will at least attract attention to the possibilities.

After a computer video course on genetics given by UCLA Professor Robert Goldberg, I find there may be ways of identifying disruption of genes by toxins ingested as food additives that will lead to the causes of many of the unknown caused problems mentioned above. If excess filtering of toxins with running exercise eliminates enough toxins for good health, this is another encouragement for older non-runners to take up our sport. It is also a new method of identifying the toxins that then can be illuminated from our diets.

Lap 45 ~ Sexology

Perhaps it's my age or my upbringing, but I am not comfortable in discussing sex publically. Did I mention previously that women runners are advised not to make eye contact with male runners? That is good advice.

To elaborate on that is once again to mention my personal experience. In the period I have called my "metamorphosis" when I thought the exercise of running was the cause of my euphoria and improved feeling in general, I stopped pursuing the reason. In retrospect I now believe cleansing my system of collected "stuff" stored due to insufficient exercise and, thus, inadequate blood circulation was the cause. Along with the exercise came an increased blood flow that resulted in the "cleansing." Whatever the cause was, it resulted in a dramatic improvement in my sexual activity.

I cannot verify that conclusion with any statistical information, but I can at least wonder if all runners are sexier than non-runners without taking all the medication to improve their sex lives that non-runners are advised to take in advertisements.

Once again, one day when you ask your doctor if you might take a prescription to enhance your sexual activity, he may say, "Yes or you can take up running to do it without medication." Once again, start running before you have a need to.

Lap 46 ~ Inherited Health

It seems to me that when running I have a clearer head than while at rest. Here are a few thoughts about running, thought of while running. One day I decided if I am called on to lecture about the subject or to brag about my book, as I approach the podium after being introduced, I will purposely fall down. On arising and speaking, I will admit to the charade as an introduction to my talk. It is an example of the fact that to be human, we are all born with a skeletal system but runners keep the system healthy.

There are many traits we humans have that make us human that are not found in other creatures as far as science has discovered such as hate, love, talking, laughing and crying, although some creatures seem to almost accomplish some of those traits. Another trait we are all able to enjoy that few other animals can equal is running distances. A horse cannot equal us and an antelope cannot do it. Mankind can run down almost all other animals. Exceptions may be some breeds of dogs and wolves.

Assuming readers accept "theories" such as gravity and evolution, is the fact that, for survival, being able to run for distances suggests another "theory" for humans. I think so and would like to explore reasons as a result of publications of anthropologists. Out of the jungle to walk and to talk and to become humanoid had to affect humans in unknown ways.

We can surmise that early man gathered in small groups around campfires with fossil evidence. We can assume man was not only a hunter but a prey of roving giant cats or other beasts. We can assume that with the advent of controlling fire, dangerous beasts would be repelled from a camp at night until the fires dwindled when another factor may enter the study. Apparently man has always required sleep and a dog would bark when sensing danger as an alarm long before man could be aware of the danger. More about this later.

With the canines entering the picture, it seems logical to me that the tamest of the wolf-like animals found that by following man on hunting excursions would result in leftovers for the animals. Gradually, the dog would join in the chase.

It has recently been expressed that man may have eaten carrion as could dogs following humans. There may have been times when humans killed and ate the camp following dogs but it may have eventually evolved that humans found some dogs to be so valuable in the hunt they became protectors of the hunting companions.

Lap 47 ~ Wolf Ancestor

This concerns the various traits of the modern-day wolf that could have been of survival help to man when early man had come out of the African forest. The landscape of the location of the group would determine which trait would be of value in a dog following the hunters. If the hunting area was open space as prairies are, a sight-hunting dog would be of most help and we find the necessary traits in Greyhound type dog camp-followers. If the group was in a thick brushy area, the pointing traits that have evolved to the likes of the pointing breeds would be of most benefit. The hound traits of trailing one particular animal would be useful in driving game animals to exhaustion. You, the reader, can elaborate on other speculations.

I am told that even today there are over 150 "tribal" groups scattered over Africa. If thousands of years ago, our evolving ancestors did first accommodate dog-like animals and gradually utilize them for the necessary means of gaining food, that could have contributed to survival that without working together neither might have survived.

In addition rather than the survival of the fittest, man may have played a major role in which type dog was permitted to survive. It would still be survival of the fittest but the fittest according to man's desires and not to nature alone.

For me it seems probable and not only possible that man

required dogs for either man or dog to survive to come out of Africa to populate the earth.

Lap 48 ~ More Enlightenment

Just when I thought all my ideas on the subject of senior running had been written and all loose ends had been carefully tucked in and the package tied with a big bow I decided I was wrong. I recalled a running shirt slogan someone suggested, "ONCE I THOUGHT I WAS WRONG BUT I WAS MISTAKEN."

While running on our new Brattleboro Union High School track, I was pondering on a remark made by so many students of human physical culture that the more exercise for humans, the healthier we are. Again that haunting word, "Why?" It suddenly came to me. The more exercise, the more sweat! Of course. I have mentioned that sweat is similar to urine. At least one book has been written about encouraging sweating as a human medical procedure.

My father had been on peritoneal dialysis for three years before he died and during that time I had hired a Russian veterinarian, Rostislaw Harchenko (he changed his name to Rosty Arch), who had immigrated here but had poor use of English. Hearing about my father's case, he brought me a book written in Russian with illustrations of wrapping a patient in woolen blankets and exposing him to heat with the resulting soaking of blankets with sweat. The theory was that by the heat and sweat, toxins would be eliminated that compromised kidneys could not eliminate. And there is more to that thought later in the book.

Of course! That observation is in keeping with my theories about running as exercise resulting in the body ridding itself of waste materials that could be responsible for some of the problems of mankind that have no other explanation as to cause. The toxins may be eliminated in internal organs, sweat, tears and saliva as well as in the urine and stool.

Here is an avenue of research in need of investigation. Perhaps absorbing patches of material to soak up sweat could be analyzed to determine the nature of toxins in the sweat. Then perhaps, those toxins could be eliminated from our diets without the need of excess exercise.

Here I have to wonder about the amount of exercise that is ideal for aging seniors. The question of whether the exercise of a 5k run in a 65 year old may be equal to the exercise of a 10k run for a 20 year old. Perhaps we seniors need more exercise to equal the good exercise does for juniors. Don't you wish you were young enough to start some of the research suggested in this book? I do.

Lap 49 ~ A Downfall?

You will enjoy talking with just about anyone who comes out to a race. When you see a runner waiting for the race to start, asking one question as an ice breaker works every time. "Have you ever fallen down in a race or in training?" Only a very few of those asked will reply in the negative. Many immediately point to old scars usually near their knees. One replied, "Have I ever and I took three guys and a girl out with me. What a pile up!" Usually that question results in information as to the date and location of a race, as well as the reason, and most claim rough pavement or unexpected curbing as the cause. Only one claimed a serious injury resulted. He actually fractured his wrist. Science tells us that exercise strengthens bone and that may be the reason so few runners' falls are serious.

You may find as I have that most runners take pleasure in talking about races they have enjoyed and why. Soon you will find yourself in that category, too.

One 5k race I ran combined paved roads and through the woods. About halfway, the race director was waiting and ran with me. He warned about roots and stones on the trail that I was well aware of. Then he mentioned areas covered with the groundcover, myrtle (periwinkle). I glanced up to look and tripped on a root and down I went. The following year running the same race, I fell for no reason I could identify and ran in with a bloody knee. Neither incidence was a problem for my running.

Once again, TIE especially where there may be obstacles.

Lap 50 ~ Who Are All These People?

The racing scene is so interesting to me, I quite regularly pause to look at the members of the assembling crowd. Many I have conversed with off and on. In a way there seems to be sameness about the group due perhaps to the running attire but a great difference in individuals. Many are lanky of any height. Then there are the males and females with heavier thighs and muscular legs than most and somehow unlikely appearing runners who consistently win awards. There is one feature of all such groups often of 300 to 400 or more. Everybody has a sort of an aura of good health. Everyone you glance at and note whether standing or walking, talking or not, everybody seems to be in good physical condition. Perhaps that has something to do with the attitude of so many. The crowd is uniformly upbeat with always laughter here and there.

Once again I ask myself, why? I think it is the personal satisfaction of knowing they are ready to do something they have prepared for and therefore will enjoy. Perhaps subconsciously they are personally involved with most of their friends who could not equal their effort because of never having discovered the satisfaction with the resulting better health.

Recently before a race I looked around at the varied members of the crowd and thought about individuals. There were teachers, doctors, lawyers, artists, nurses and all sorts of business folks and all kinds of workers of all ages. A charming group with any one of whom I would like to start up a conversation. It seems to me we all have a lot in common.

None smoke and few take drugs such as alcohol other than socially and most are not overweight. I suspect most are careful of their diets and all are concerned with keeping in some degree of good physical shape. Strange but in over ten years of small talk before and after races, I have heard only one so called swear word and that was from my friend, Dr. Art Snyder, who has taken up the interest in providing me with water and a shoulder to grab at the conclusion of many races we both have run. That may sound like some sort of snob appeal exists with runners but just the opposite is the case. That kind of mix of members of society doesn't exist in most groups. Running seems to be a leveling agent. Even with large numbers and ample refreshments, grounds are never littered with trash after races. Is it a special mindset for runners?

After a 5k race on a warm day, out of the crowd of runners stepped Connecticut's popular State Attorney General Blumenthal, wet with sweat as we all were to congratulate me. He has since been elected a Senator from Connecticut. Many outstanding notables are regular runners. Of course, past presidents Bush and Carter have been runners. So to join our group will find you in good company most of the time.

Running is truly a democratic sport. A good example of the popularity of the sport is the yearly New England high school cross-country championship race. Thousands of families and friends gather to watch and cheer for hundreds of high school runners who attack a 5k course. Such an event demonstrated to me the thousands out for such a festive occasion did not represent the lost generation so often mentioned about our present day youth. Here was the future of our country and it seemed to me that it would be in good hands.

Lap 51 ~ Late Bloomer

At a recent race along Long Island Sound, the winner was an M40 runner, Joel Bender of Bedford, Connecticut, and I had a talk with him. He was aware that I had started running late in life and he wanted me to know he had been an average runner in his younger days but had given it up until recently when he restarted our sport. Since restarting he has become faster and faster as he trained in spite of his aging. There is an old rule of thumb that after seriously starting, runners reach their prime after 10 years of running. For me it was after five years when I was awarded the distinction of being "outstanding athlete" for the year 2004 in my 80-84 age class. Dorothy, my late wife, said, "Yes, but that's only in the United States." That award was by the previously mentioned USATF, the largest group representing Track and Field in our land. I wonder if some of the runners of old who have given up the sport restarted, would excel in their new senior age groups? I believe they would be surprised at their latent ability. How can they be encouraged?

At that race I made a discovery about which I have hesitated mentioning without more data. I have asked hundreds of runners if they had headaches and I found that when a young runner said he had occasional headaches while running. After posting the above as a blog on my computer, Ilsa Barkley, W60, an excellent runner tells me she has had headaches off and on for years even in the clean Oregon air and running. That brings forth another question, are people with migraine headaches runners? It would be interesting if those with that debilitating problem were never runners.

Lap 52 ~ Race Names

When your fingers are wandering idly over the computer keys, hunting for a scheduled race, you might be confused by race names. With the enthusiasm of some race organizers and directors, many races seem to take on a life of their own. Many have been around for many years. There are plenty to go around. Here is a brief sampling from my area while in Connecticut and the list could become a volume if other areas of the country were included. Most are 5k races but there is a sampling of longer races, too.

Tradition, Resolution, Sweetheart, Shamrock, April Fool's, Spirit of Spring, Feed the Need, Run for Your Life, Bunny Boggle, River Run, Clamdigger, Daffodil Festival, Run for Rescue, Seaside Shuffle, Sprint Into Spring, Polar Bear, Leprechaun, Spring Equinox, Minuteman, Lightfoot, Irish Festival, Chilly-Chili, Jingle Bell . . . and that's only a sample.

Lap 53 ~ What Trophies?

The older we runners get, the more trophies we win. I asked one fairly good runner what he does with his trophies. "Trophies? I've been running for over 20 years and never have won a trophy." Others tell me they donate them to the local high school and others give them to a running store to donate to the most worthy cause.

Since I started running at 80 years of age, I rarely run without winning (or should I say being given) a trophy. If not a running figure, ribbons with medallions or sometimes just ribbons.

My good wife used to suggest that I dust my trophies so I wrap each in a disposable plastic bag and fill boxes to be used in a special way. I am leaving a stipend of money to my coach to use as a special memorial race with little or no entry fee and that somehow encourages older runners. There are already plenty of trophies for the first three winners in each age group and sex. It seems to me it is the least I can do to repay a fraction of the pleasure I have had during my running "career."

There is also a collection of perhaps 100 T-shirts with slogans printed on the backs. I would like to have the collection given out to the first 100 or so who register for such a memorial race.

Some trophies are presented by attractive females. I

make it a policy of asking, "Don't I get a kiss?" The results are consistently good.

In a race after my 90th birthday in Monroe, Connecticut, I was given a trophy larger than the winner of the race and that winner had finished the 5k 30 minutes before me. Race directors are delighted to have seniors of both sexes run in their races.

Lap 54 ~ Fountain of Youth?

We all know we slow down a little more every year but there is an important objective for all runners and that is to slow down the slowing down. How to do it? I do think I would be even slower if I didn't work out regularly. I have tried all sorts of formulas such as the interval running and fartleks (Scandinavian training system with bursts of speed) and long runs that for me are five miles at this time. I decided I am in reasonable shape and did back-to-back 5k's on the same day with no ill effects. Early in 2006, I decided to do 5k's daily for seven days of training. I followed that with two days rest and ran a 5k organized race. I did not improve my time by a second. My latest effort is to rest two or three days after every serious effort. While doing the seven 5k's and noting the times, it was remarkable to find that several were within 10 seconds of the others. All that concentrated work seemed fruitless until I realized it kept me from slowing down more than otherwise and, a week later with no workouts, my time in a 5k was my best of the year.

Be your own scientist and experiment and if you find a better idea, let me hear from you.

Lap 55 ~ Take a Trip with Me

Do you like to travel? Even if you dislike traveling, come along on this trip for the fun of it. Bring friends and an enemy. Hold your palm up in front of you and what do you see? I see a pink palm and assume yours is, too. Do you wonder why? Another question. That's an easy one to answer because we all learn that blood is red and through the skin the hemoglobin gives skin that pink color. Thousands of microscopic cells in percentage of numbers most of which are red cells are responsible. I'll include an enemy we can call a toxin for an example on our trip. Where is one of those red cells and the enemy going and how rapidly do they travel? Let's say it's a fairly dark red cell and it's traveling in a minute vessel called a capillary. It has lost much of its oxygen and is being conducted back toward the lungs to get recharged. It heads toward a vein to finally enter the heart, from which it is sent promptly to the lungs to get recharged with oxygen along with the toxin and then back to your heart to your finger as arterial blood. Right? Yes, however, it may not go directly back. It may go to the kidneys and then back to the heart to the lungs and out toward your finger, but may make a detour through the liver and then back to the heart and lungs before it gets back to your finger.

Take a siesta from our trip to wonder about some other things taking place. In the first place, that red blood cell does not work forever. It has a life expectation of let's say 30 days. It has to be eliminated. Our immune system is involved as it is with any unwanted bacteria and other stuff like the unwanted toxin for good health. It just may be the toxin we have eaten came in food with ingredients that the system takes five or six circuits through our blood vascular apparatus before it is illuminated. It may also be called a poison.

With so many places for the toxin as well as our red cell to go before returning to our finger, I doubt either of the two will ever return. They could go through all our internal organs including our sense organs such as eyes, nose, ears and even under finger and toe nails. The possibilities are almost infinite. You might like to know, evidence in science is undecided as to the accuracy of the 30-day life expectancy of the red blood cell, and it and the nature of the toxin and resistance of our bodies must depend to some extent on the activity (metabolic rate) of individuals.

Does that sound complicated? To say complicated is putting it mildly. There are white cells and platelets and the fluid all in our blood vascular system all aiding and concerned with the housekeeping necessary for good health. All that to suggest that exercise is important to circulate the blood to have it cleaned of the sorts of stuff including the toxin that may not be welcome in a healthy you or me.

We know that some substances may accumulate gradually over the years to slowly damage us. It seems to me that such a situation may be common and never discovered during a lifetime, but since humans are born with the ability to run, it may be reasonable that running or a similar exercise is necessary for the increased circulation needed to circulate the blood enough to rid a system of the bad stuff. It is with this reasoning that I am urging you to quit lazing around and to get out and run for your life and, as I have said repeatedly, you will feel the improvement early in your training to be an enjoyment unappreciated by indolent others.

Lap 56 ~ What's Going On?

Someone must have said, "It's fun to be fooled but it's more fun to know." This will scratch the surface of what happens when you jog or run. Think about it. Every step by putting one foot down, you ever so lightly jar your brain. Not enough to give anyone I have heard about a headache but when you think about it, there is that slight jolt. So what? Tell the likes of Sam Harris, a brain neurologist and he may light up and think of the chemicals in our brains that have profound effect on whatever it is to be normal. Science is making astounding discoveries about brain chemistry and that jolting may have a lot to do with the claim that those who exercise most are healthiest.

It's obvious that in the chest, the heart must pump blood to nourish the needs of our moving parts and the lungs must filter the air and exchange bad for good where it is recirculated through our bodies and that is well recognized, but below our diaphragm things are also happening that seem just as remarkable as above.

Coach Chuck suggested that the liver, gall bladder and stomach are neatly packed together with the spleen, pancreas and small and large intestines along with two kidneys and genitals pretty much filling up that space. So what? Well, think of the fact that with every jogging or running step, all those abdominal organs are also subjected to that jarring with each step. Even with those who run for marathon distances, I have never heard of any runner having had even a stomach ache. Rarely a stitch in the side but never a stomach ache.

In 1943 when I graduated from the School of Veterinary Medicine at Auburn University, we were told the liver had at least 200 functions and today that figure by Wikipedia in my computer has risen to "over 1,000." The pressure of jogging or running does not seem to be unfavorable to the liver, but it may well be found that the slight thumping is helpful to all those organs.

I mention the above because when running or jogging, I often think about such things and have mixed feelings. On the one hand, I may smile thinking that I can do something that millions could do but most don't. Then a sadness descends as I wonder about the better health and happiness millions of couch potatoes could experience if only they were made aware they are capable but don't realize it. So perhaps this book should be called an experiment in education. Time will tell.

Next will be an ego trip.

Lap 57 ~ Don't Give Up the Ship

Now let's come home from our trip and bring our egos along. One reason for the lack of large numbers of older runners may be our egos. It seems to me that we oldies think we have "earned" a little respect and consideration in our maturing years. At a recent race at the Harbor Yard in Bridgeport, Connecticut, I was straining away during a 5k race when a little girl held by the hand of her father passed me. I watched her skip and leave her father to "tight-rope" walking along the curb still faster than my pace. I was told later her name was Kirsten Johnston and her dad, Robert. I did pass them from time to time until we came to an area with two-foot-high orange colored cones along the way. Kirsten left her father and played leapfrog over all 20 or so cones as her father hurried to keep up. She was hurrying to the end of the race that both reached long before I could make it. I marveled at the dancing, skipping, hopping as well as running so much faster than I that I wondered if I should give up as a hopelessly slow runner. Then it came to me, I wondered how fast she and her dad would be when 87 years old and I decided at that point to keep on trying, ego or no ego. Perhaps I should print on a running shirt, "DON'T GIVE UP THE SHIP" or "NEVER, NEVER, NEVER, NEVER give up." TIE, yes, but don't give up.

Lap 58 ~ Prejudice

Prejudice is, to me, an ugly word. It seems strange that such an uplifting sport as ours finds so many guilty of discrimination. When we mature runners see an entry blank for a race that states blatantly 60+ as the upper-age group, we are staring at prejudice against older runners. I've seen it with a church as a beneficiary of the funds raised. When each of us is confronted with such discrimination, we should at least send a letter stating, "No thanks."* I would think even the youngsters in their 50's would respond similarly as they soon will be faced with the same insult. We all should encourage a boycott of such a race as well as a letter of protest. The point being, why should we in our 80's have to compete with those youngsters in their 70's? Perhaps it is due to the fact that a large percent of runners are under 60 where the entry fee is the hallmark of success. Or perhaps the directors concentrate on the youngsters due to the scarcity of us mature runners. Let's all work on increasing the numbers of senior runners.

As of this date in our area, the three busiest race directors have recognized older runners. I mentioned Marty Schaivonne before. He was soon followed by Joe Riccio in recognizing older runners. Joe, who is also a runner, has become a personal friend. Not infrequently, he meets me at

* See Appendix 5, page 154

about a half mile before the finish of races to give encouragement. In one race he awarded me a trophy for being the oldest runner in the race. John Bysiewicz is the race director for the New Haven Championship 20k Labor Day Race and many other races, who also recognizes older runners.

Lap 59 ~ About Speed

About speed: I have asked many experienced runners how to increase speed. One seemed to make sense. He said speed is determined by the length of time you run with both feet off the ground. Now that sounds reasonable, doesn't it? I thought so until one day my coach-son in Maine emailed me that he had a fast high school walker who had broken the school record for the fast walk of the mile in just under six minutes. In fast walking, one rule is that you never walk with both feet off the ground at the same time. So what involves speed in running? It seems to me it is how fast you can move your legs and, until someone makes me a better suggestion, I'll consider how older runners can move our legs faster.

It may be that at 90 years of age, I am no longer able to run with more than one foot off the ground and I believe when into our 80's, most of us find it to be so.

Fast walking and slow running have much in common but if you analyze each, you will appreciate that quite different muscles are used for walking as compared to those used for running or jogging.

You may experience running, even when slow, that it seems to be a fast pace when most everyone else in some races pass you. In reality, yours may be actually fast for your age group. That's part of the mystique of senior running.

Lap 60 ~ Diet and Other Trivia

Here is a simple formula for a diet that cannot miss. When next you meet a class runner from Kenya, ask him what he eats and follow his diet exactly. It seems to me that there are no human experts on what to eat as compared to the advice veterinarians advise their clients for infra human animals. If you have lived to a satisfactory senior age, it is obvious you had to have eaten with common sense and that's the best diet.

Years ago our family attended swimming meets at Yale University where an Australian swimmer, Schulhamer, I think was his name, set many distance records for the Yale team. On reading about him, I was amazed to find he was a vegetarian and ate only vegetables and not even eggs or dairy products. I recall an appropriate quote for that situation. "There are many roads to the top of the mountain but when you get there the view is the same."

As far as when to eat, there may be some common sense about not loading your stomach too close to when you sally forth for a training run or for when the gun goes off. Plan to eat after training or racing.

I drink a glass of orange juice an hour or more before going out to exercise but most of those I ask when to eat say, eat a light meal before a race or training period. We know something about blood sugar and for some it is a more important consideration than for others. It appears that runners eat a lot of bananas. They digest easily and are rich in potassium, the bananas that is.

How in the world did our ancestors survive without knowing how much of what they should have to eat to run well? Of course, they did not know even as little as we know. Our ancestors ate fruit when it was around or the carcass of game with little else until it was gone, when they no doubt ate of the harvest available once they learned how to plant and reap.

In nature the varied diets of all sorts of living creatures have been recorded by scientists who noted stomach contents in describing them. I can find that sort of knowledge has never been recorded for the superior creature in relation to running because, perhaps until Darwin, even scientists did not consider humans to be in the animal kingdom.

Lap 61 ~ More Diet

There was a time during which vitamins that had been recently discovered played a part in a condition called "growing pains" in adolescent children. The human medical profession told mothers that their children needed extra vitamins A and D to be healthy. I recall coming home from grammar school and my friends having to get their cod liver oil. My mother did not go with that fad but many mothers overdid the vitamins and often gave a tablespoon of the vile stuff to their children. A significant number of the recipients developed what was called, "growing pains." Some of my friends had such pains, often in knees so severe that they went so far as using crutches to get around with less pain. Today our milk is fortified with adequate amounts of vitamin D. I would think the vitamins suggested to be taken once a day would be adequate if taken once a week. The cod liver oil was stopped as were the growing pains.

Scientific research indicates that too much of some other vitamins some people take today can be inadvisable. Moderation always seems appropriate. In considering diets of our ancestors, remember their life expectancy was somewhere over 35 years.

So the real answer is to eat what has agreed with you since it has sustained you all your life and use common sense as to how long an interval is best to digest your food before a race or workout. Appreciate the fact that most of your nutrition to be healthy was eaten often months before the exercise we are talking about.

The following statements seem to make sense to me:

- Sugar contains half the calories as an equal amount of fat.
- High sugar consumers are more likely to be slimmer.
- Exercise reduces levels of sugar rapidly but of fat slowly.
- Research suggests a high-fat, high-energy intake with a sedentary lifestyle are two main causes of weight gain.
- A combination of carbohydrate diet including sugar with running can assist in normal weight.

I have never heard of a runner who disliked ice cream.

Lap 62 ~ Outhouses and Salt

When I was a kid, a friend and I took an old car on a 10,000-mile trip out west and, during that trip, we went to see Hoover Dam where it was 115 in the shade and there was no shade. We were told that the workers were given canteens with salt water in them to start the day because so many workers were passing out from the salt lost in sweating. When I run in hot weather, I sweat. I like salt. Quite suddenly, there were articles all about restricting salt intake. I recalled the Hoover Dam incident and then heard that about 18 percent of older people are sensitive to salt. I was swilling special drinks for athletes and noted there was little salt in them. More recently, the need for salt for many of us put salt back in the athletic drinks.

A side note about special drinks. I was having to get up at night to pee. I had never done that before and thought it must have been the amount of H_2O I was drinking. On reading labels, I found citric acid (a preservative) in most all the drinks, so I visited our Ag Station in New Haven and the head chemist informed me that citric acid is a diuretic (makes for frequent urinating). I stopped the drinks with citric acid as well as all sorts of pastries containing it and no longer have to get up nights.

Perhaps I can be accused of having an inordinate interest in privies or outhouses or portable potties. When I had beagles for a hobby, the objective was to raise them to win in field trials. To have a field trial sanctioned, the American Kennel Club required each club to have toilet accommodations. The clubs are all located in areas far from city facilities and there were many clubs in our country. The State of Pennsylvania had over 200 such when I wrote a book about that sport. So, the AKC has photos of all the privies located where field trials occurred and, I presume, that it is the largest collection of privy pictures in the country and, perhaps, the world. With organized running races, facilities must be provided and the lines are awesome just before a running event.

If you anticipate a need as so many do, plan ahead to locate them and to utilize those symbols of civilization. In spite of all the preparations, it is not unusual to see a runner run off the course and behind an obstacle during a race. It seems to me that cemeteries are preferred. That can be a major problem for one of the fair sex but it shouldn't be.

In hot weather, it should be obvious that it may be advisable to drink immediately before a race as it is embarrassing to have to have two people in white coats carry you to a shady area for water and/or salt lost by your efforts. During many races, one or two "water holes" have volunteers handing paper cups of water to runners passing by. I suggest, if it's warm weather, you should imbibe.

I know of no scientific studies concerning drinks for athletes other than water and salt in moderation.

Lap 63 ~ A Marathon? Forget It

For beginning runners up to your 70's, you could aspire to run in a marathon or for non-runners who have given up on the sport they enjoyed years ago, perhaps you would like to consider a marathon, but I write this as an older runner who started at 80 years of age and for me a marathon has to be a spectator sport.

There are about as many training schedules to prepare for a marathon as there are running books in the library describing them. Many start out with a six-month training period. At the other end of the spectrum, there are those who want bragging rights for running in a marathon in every state in a year and others who are satisfied in running in one every week in one year.

Getting back to reality, I will get around to telling you about a half marathon I ran in with Coach Chuck and another, but for me to get in shape to run in a 5k race is as marathoners do for a marathon. The overwhelming majority of runners I know quietly bathe in the light of knowing about their own personal accomplishments. That has to be a bright light and a wonderful feeling that you can enjoy, too. *Come Jog with Me.*

Many older marathoners walk more than half the race. I will not dwell on such races and if you care to, look for other books to fill your needs. I have never run in a full marathon.

Lap 64 ~ Proof of the Puddin'

Somebody said it couldn't be done. Perhaps they have not met Barbara Jordan. Neither have I, but I've read about her. That young woman runs as a W70 (70-year-old woman) contestant in many organized races as a winner. She teaches exercise at the University of Vermont. At her tender age, she competes in many organized races. It seems to me that if she can do what she does in her 70-year-old class, almost everyone her age should be able to at least run even without attempting to set records as she does. As good as the Vermont air is, that is not the reason. The main reason she can run is that she tries. Don't you wonder if you might at least try? Please do.

Then there is another example of a senior excelling and his name is Bob Hewitt of Oregon. He excels in most events in track and field and the reason he is so outstanding in his M75 class is not the excellent air in Oregon, but because at age 65 he tried organized events 10 years ago. Doesn't that send you a message?

For the year 2010, the USATF Association designated Judge Ralph Maxwell of South Dakota as "Athlete of the Year" for his setting records with most events he enters in his age group. His is the 90-94 age group, the same as mine. We have to say, "Hats off" to the retired judge.

I mentioned previously 30 million runners in our land

who run at least once a week, have you considered seriously making it 30,000,001? An incentive could be that if you do you may result in being better at it than 50 percent of runners who have enjoyed the sport all their lives. That assumes that you will become part of the 50 percent of those who will be better, rather than the 50 percent who will be below average. The joker here is that it makes little difference which group you will find yourself in, because you will feel so improved in your own health and attitude it will not matter.

Perhaps competition is part of the human makeup but at our ages, although it may be pleasant to excel at anything, if the activity is fun then just running becomes excelling.

Lap 65 ~ Running With Pain?

In many running magazines,* running with pain is mentioned from time to time. Now at my tender age, I have to admit I don't enjoy pain. During the first few years of running I had my share of injuries. Knees, Achilles tendon, hamstring, thick wallet disease, and others not readily described in the books. It is true there was pain and I did run gently until the pain subsided and that took a while for the Achilles, but now and for five years all pain has been a thing of the past.

I asked Coach Dickerson if he ever ran with pain and he surprised me by saying, "I run with pain every race I run." As far as I am concerned, there may be a problem with definition. I try what I think is my best but I never feel pain no matter how hard I try. Not infrequently, I have to grab hold of a person at the finish to prevent my falling down, but pain? No. I can't call it that and if pain were a constant problem, I don't think I could enjoy it as I do. So when you read of pain, don't consider it a reason to forgo the pleasure of fun running, just TIE.

Thinking of pain reminds me of a time long ago when I broke a leg skiing on Mt. Mansfield here in Vermont. Did you know there is always snow at Stowe? In a hospital bed in Morrisville, Vermont, after the bones had been screwed back in place, a nurse asked me if I felt much pain. I was in great pain and told her so. She commented, "You should try having a baby." That ended my complaining about pain.

* See Appendix 9, page 165

Lap 66 ~ Running Publicity

For a sport of 30,000,000 participants, why is there not more recognition? More public relations effort? There is a good answer; it's not a spectator sport. Runners are numerous only at the start and then we trickle in and only the winners are of interest to the press. The winners cross the finish line and that's the end of the event. Marathons with cameras every mile or so, and with the huge number of participants, recognize only the leaders and they because many locals are mixed in the crowd, although usually not individually recognized. Often super-human efforts on the part of hero men and women are of little interest unless someone can alert the press as to why the effort is exceptional enough to mention.

Unlike 5k races, in marathons little is news about age-related results, only the winners, both men and women. That may seem remarkable, until you get personally involved and discover that recognition is the least important reason for running.

Perhaps there is a light at the end of you entering the competition where you may be first in your class and set some records and the running world will be informed. I hope so and if it happens, tell them I sent you.

Lap 67 ~ Special Track Meets

If you happen to be a resident of the Solace for Retirement Rest Home, you may find new runners like yourself in similar establishments giving running a try. Have your physical director arrange abbreviated track meets. Such events could be around a block in your neighborhood for one race and around another block at another rest home at a later date. You could talk with the Town Fathers and Mothers for help in having a town-wide yearly race for each age group of both sexes over 65. Don't overlook the high school or college running track. You can bet on it that such an event would make the news and be great fun. I'll run with you if you let me know in advance. There are all kinds of extras at such an event, such as having only grandchildren passing out the water. Or great-grandchildren, come to think of it. Add prizes for the grandchildren of the oldest grandparents winning an age group and those children may well grow into champion track stars. Moreover, what a great influence for those children.

Lap 68 ~ New England 65+ Runners Club

As an example of something going on in the running world, the New England 65+ Runners Club is a good example with one possible exception. Just about every person mentioned has been an established runner. Most for real long distances and most are properly acknowledged as runners who are continuing to record outstanding performances. They hold one 5k all-age gathering with the sprinkling of ancients among many fine and playful younger contestants.

Once a year they hold an annual luncheon which, because of time and distance, I have never attended. The group has a healthy steady growth record and is important to support. The one exception is, it seems to me, that their publications should try to attract more of the higher end of the 65+ age group. There is something special about the fellowship of runners in general and still something very special about the fellowship of us real old runners.

Watch for more and more similar groups and support them for not only your own good, but for that of our fellow runners and most particularly of the new ones. This club is in the Boston area, where the numbers of races on any weekend in good weather is awesome. I predict the same will happen on our West Coast, if it hasn't already. That's just a little more frosting on your cake. Join in.

Lap 69 ~ Level the Playing Field

Can an argument be made that for older runners, the playing field in organized races is not as equal as it is for younger runners? Can a case be made that it could be called prejudice again?

Now let's say records are kept of the best time for each age group on each established race course. Say a 5k race had 16 minutes for the most fleet age group and that was the course record. The fastest runner of the day in a race was a 20 year old who ran it in 15:40. That is 20 seconds under the 16-minute race record. In the 70-year age group, the course record for a 70 year old was 35 minutes and s/he ran it in 34:30. That time was 30 seconds under the track record. That 70 year old would be the race winner for that day, provided no other age group winner had a better time. It's called leveling the playing field.

I'm sure many have suggested similar solutions to the problem of fairness to all age runners, and I think we might find many runners reentering the sport and making interesting waves. We know the sport is growing every year and that idea would add a fairness that could entice many wonderful athletes back in the sport. Moreover, it might produce outstanding runners from those starting the sport over the age of 65 who might set records.

Perhaps you and I will live long enough to see it happen nationwide.

Lap 70 ~ Hitting on Her

Even if you are not interested in one of the other sex for romantic reasons, you may be happily surprised to find one interested in you at races or training. With others trying my prescription with you, you will find many enjoying the opportunity of gathering together to run or to jog. With others with the same objectives of better health and happiness, life takes on an interesting new dimension.

When runners gather regularly, friendships develop and I told my daughter, Lee, my keeper, about two young 70-year-old women runners and especially about one. Lee said, "Dad, you're hitting on her." I had never heard the term before and asked what she meant. It seems to me that to be nice to those you admire does not have to be "hitting on them."

You may start alone to jog as I did, but when you find others of like mind it is more interesting and opens the way to togetherness even among strangers. Try it and prove me right. If running with others results in matrimony, even if against your plans, blame it on me and perhaps I'll come to your wedding.

Lap 71 ~ Do Runners Live Longer?

We often hear that runners may not live longer than the average but we die healthier. I intend to attempt to prove that runners do actually live longer than the average human. This is only one reason among many.

For 2006 it was stated by one medical report that 750,000 cases of injuries occurring in and around the home to seniors over 65 years of age were serious enough to be admitted to hospitals. Most of the injuries involved fractured bones.

Hospital-related infections are obscenely common in even the best hospitals and the fatality rates of such infections are also obscene. By running and maintaining healthy bones we runners, therefore, have many fewer injuries and, therefore, fewer hospital adventures and it follows that we have fewer hospital-related infections. Q.E.D. (quad erat demonstrandum), few fatalities.

Incidentally during my 10 years of running, I have fallen at least 16 times and gotten up and continued each time with only an injured pride.

That argument only considers bone fractures and it is a given that those who really do exercise regularly are healthier than others.

One human surgeon was heard to remark that he prefers to operate on runners because they rarely contract hospital-related infections.

Lap 72 ~ Cherry Picking the Research

We all should think scientifically about our activities in life and not accept statements by revelation. I find the need of proof and proof I can accept as valid usually by the source. So I have decided to cherry pick the information favorably and unfavorably expressed about running as exercise. In combing the literature, almost all the results are favorable so it will appear that I have chosen only the good proof as you will see.

Study after study has been published on specific reasons for real exercise I have mentioned, as running is. At least 10 years ago, scientists at the Salk Institute in California reported that exercise stimulates the creation of brand new nerve cells in the brain. Wow, now that's good news when you hear about the loss of brain cells with aging with Alzheimer's disease. Of course, science recognizes that new discoveries that answer questions result in more questions. So we might like to know if there is less Alzheimer's disease in older runners. My mother died with it. Could she still be alive had she learned to *Come Jog with Me* when she was 65 years of age?

I have to ask the same about my wife who died at 93 with a heart problem. She had been an Adirondack mountain climber when young and if she had been interested in my plea to you to *Come Jog with Me*, would we still be together?

Human medical report after report claim that real exercise results in less heart disease.

Lap 73 ~ The Invisible Runner

In this book you may notice I am trying to convince all readers to at least try my prescription for an immediate improvement to their lives, as well as paving the way for a smoother and longer life. At the same time I am trying to address as many of the reasons or excuses that a reader can offer for not attempting to improve her- or himself. I have challenged with all sorts of sincere and scientifically proven reasons to accept the insurance policy.* Another possible consideration came to mind while running that may be your excuse.

It may be that some people may think they do not want to be seen doing something as outrageous as running at their advanced age. I have a solution for you. Be an invisible runner. That is to anyone who may recognize you. Tell the family members that you are going out for a walk somewhere where you are least apt to be seen by anyone who you think might think you are an emergency.

If you think your anatomy is a problem such as men with large waist lines and women with big boobs, phone a running store a distance away from home, of course, and discover how cooperative they will be. When you are outfitted properly, go to a remote flat surface area where you can follow the instructions in this book and undergo a metamorphosis.

* See Lap 5, Page 10

Turn into a runner. It doesn't matter how poor a runner you may become, because the prize you will win will be a welcome surprise for you, and for me, personally, it will be the satisfaction of knowing I helped someone who will drop me a note of thanks

Lap 74 ~ Labor Day

Here is the anatomy of a special race labeled "National Championship 20k Road Race" New Haven, Connecticut, that becomes a special place for Labor Day. Not only do about 6,000 runners congregate on the New Haven Green but their friends, relatives and have-been runners and others just to watch and perhaps cheer. Drop by any year and enjoy it yourself. There is a 5k race simultaneously.

Yours truly decided to run in the 20k race and I invited my son-coach, Chuck, to run, too. He accepted and for what he thought might be a good reason. I suspect he thought that at my age I might be in need of special assistance.

Preparation for the race consisted of consulting with Coach Dickerson many months prior to it, who advised me to add a mile to my workouts once a week. Running for five miles resulted in difficulty with that fifth mile and when I graduated to six, that last mile was tough. The same was true up to and including the seventh mile of seven. Then I made myself slow down from the beginning of the nine-mile run and it was a cinch, as was mile 10. Coach told me to take it easy before the race. I'm still trying to know how to take it easy.

The same problem overtook me on that Labor Day when, with the pleasure of having my son run with me and the excitement of the event, I ran too fast in the beginning. It was a sad ending with my walking the last two miles. However I did set a record for my age group for the 20k race.

More recently, determined to run that race from beginning to end, I trained more but gave out again at the end finishing in three hours and some minutes. With about a mile and a half to go, another runner watched this old man struggling and with compassion ran by my side to the finish when I knew he could have doubled his speed with no trouble. At the end, I learned his name to be Jonathon Murphy and I am indebted to him. So many runners are special.

A few remarks about that yearly race are in order. The chairman of the huge committee overseeing the race is John Courtmanche, a class runner in his age group since he started running. The race director is John Bysiewicz, a master race director and runner, too. Along the route are numerous music makers and of course "water holes" manned by many wonderful volunteer groups. The Police Department of New Haven takes an outstanding part with so many intersections and even leading in their vehicles the likes of me when most runners have long since passed. In the 2006 race, about half a mile from the finish, the Amity High School of Woodbridge, Connecticut, Women's cross-country team with their Coach Dickerson met to run in with me. Even though I was struggling with my walking with that 45-degree angle, we received great cheers while the young women sang songs and generally made merry along the way. In that 2006 race none other than Chairman Courtmanche himself greeted me toward the end, encouraging me to "take it easy" as I approached the finish. There at the finish was my youngest daughter, Lee, and her two sons, Leon and Chuck, wishing me well.

With that kind of experience you have to not only see it but feel it to believe it. More seniors should have that opportunity. I now know with my age slowing down I will never be able to manage such a race again and I doubt any new readers my age will be able to either. Stay with the shorter races and enjoy them if you are close to my age.

I strongly urge all readers to attend such a half marathon as an audience for an uplifting memorable experience.

Lap 75 ~ Why Runners Retire

Since I have had so much pleasure in the sport of organized running the question, "Why do runners stop running?" comes to mind. One obvious problem in reaching an answer to that question is that many of those who have quit are not on earth to answer the question. However, a few volunteers are in that category and many know friends who no longer take advantage of the opportunity. Here are a collection of "reasons." Heading the list seems to be injuries. One friend has had reconstructive surgery to an ankle and several have mentioned chronic knee problems. Another curious answer was that they no longer felt the need to keep running. One senior who was an outstanding runner in days gone by said he was transferred to an area where the smog was so terrible he thought it would affect his health deleteriously. He quit. Later he moved to Vermont where the air is excellent and has not taken the sport up again.

Early one cool Sunday morning (25 degrees F) while running on the streets of Brattleboro, a car pulled out of a driveway just ahead of me. That left me in the fumes of combustion I tried not to breathe. There was no breeze to carry the foul smelling fumes away and, to my surprise, those fumes lasted for half a city block. I thought of the traffic jams and aerial views of traffic on highways everywhere and it seemed to me that it is not necessary to be a professional climatologist to know that those fumes from every car and most houses are contaminating our atmosphere perhaps beyond repair. Is there a time when it will be too late to do something about it?

Continuing the reasons for retiring, one merely said, "I got married." I asked why that had anything to do with running and he just smiled and walked away. With my late wife who was so supporting, I still wonder why that one gave it up. When I mentioned that reason, several runners mentioned that they had met women who ran during courtship and some after marriage took up running. Several had stopped and after a time started up again. Some of those had been told by a physician they would become hopeless cripples if they continued. Others were advised to run to get in and keep in shape. Several of those had been running well in their age groups until a spouse quit so they did, too.

I think the major "reasons" for giving up the sport is the loss of speed with aging. After so many of an age group are no longer running, there is less and less competition and the athlete who once felt he represented his age group well, finds most of the runners leaving him behind and it is less fun with each race.

When races are highlighted to encourage older runners, we seniors come out from distances for such a race. Such is the "Over 65 New England"* group, mentioned previously, who highlight at least one race a year in Wakefield, Mass. Take your pick and if I hear of other reasons, I'll add them for future reference.

* See Appendix 9, page 165

Lap 76 ~ Come Dream with Me

I had a vision. It was not quite like Martin Luther King's dream but for me it was a vision. So, take my hand and come with me to a new time in road racing. In the Senior Sporting Club there are many older men and women as well as lots of children. A sign at one table reads, "PREREGISTERED 65-69, 70-74, 75-79, 80-84, 85-89, and 90 and up." At another, "REGISTER TODAY. 65-74 and 75-up." What is this place and who are all these happy people?

The year is 2020 and this is the inaugural of the racing season for seniors only. So many people over 65 years of age have discovered the fun and the value of running as a hobby that there are, starting this year, 5k road races certified by the USATF. Only men and women over 65 years of age are permitted to run and no dogs on leashes or bicycles.

We are welcomed by parents and grandparents of many of the volunteers who are the children relatives of the older runners. We learn that groups of children will be along the route of the race cheering their elders and handing out paper cups of water to thirsty runner-relatives. Earlier, an ambulance from the local emergency service had driven up and would be in touch with other volunteers with cell phones along the route.

For some strange reason, many are wearing different colored socks and bright running shorts and the atmosphere is one of cheer and happiness. Recognizing a friend nearby, one runner calls out, "Hello Marge, I didn't know you were into it, too." The fun continues before, during and after the race.

Well, there is a scene you can be a part of and can check out my vision for yourself. That's if you *Come Jog with Me* now. I'll join you if I'm still around.

Lap 77 ~ More Ponderings

Mentioned previously have been thoughts while spending time running that may be unique because of the opportunity running affords. Toward the end of composing this document while on a three-mile run, my thinking was directed to what has gone on to produce me. My ancestors and yours and everybody's are responsible for the results that are us. We have inherited valor, guts, perhaps cowardice and all our mental and physical characteristics. We have an immune system that survived plagues that killed so many of our ancestors. Periods of sparse food and faulty nutrition. Floods and earthquakes, all because of either special traits or of good fortune of our ancestors are reasons. We are really each a fantastic creature.

As fantastic as that seems, the chance that each of us living here on earth is even more fantastic. Think about the millions of sperm present to fertilize one of many eggs to start the development of one individual. No two of the sperm can make duplicate individuals. Over a lifetime, think of the chance that one sperm and one of many hundreds of eggs were necessary to create every individual not only here and now but over the generations of evolution. How many ejaculations with how many billions of spermatozoa that did not fertilize an egg for you to be the only one? You are indeed unique, as am I.

With that in mind, it seems such a tragedy for any human

to be killed for any other than extreme reasons, although we treat one killing as a murder and may be horrified, we ask our military to murder and call it foreign policy and forget it. For shame.

I like to finish many of my workouts or races with the thought that this event is a tribute to my ancestors and smile. I know my parents would be proud. Wouldn't yours?

Lap 78 ~ Time to Quit

They say there is a time for everything, as the song goes, and I believe all older humans should wake up to this being the proper time. Time to quit sitting around without much exercise. Time to quit resting while really doing nothing. Time to quit spending hours with a jigsaw puzzle when you could be running. Time to quit complaining about stiffness. Time to quit taking medications when running replaces them. Time to quit adding an inch or more to your waistline yearly. It's time to quit thinking that you cannot relearn to run. Time to quit thinking that you believe running is unacceptable work. Time to quit thinking there is something bad about work.

It is really time to quit the negatives and embrace the obvious positives of getting out for your first jogging experience. The remainder of your life will be a revelation. Here, then, is another question and answer, "If for me, why not for you?"

Lap 79 ~ A New Beginning?

If you do pursue the sport of running for any reason and are a senior (over 65 or so), you may become a celebrity in demand to lecture to groups such as service clubs and others. You may find yourself written up in the news under "good news" rather than the usual depressing news that most editors find sell papers. If so, you can be an emissary of good will in encouraging other seniors to join us in fun running.

If you do enter this group, you may even save lives and or make lives more meaningful. By example, some of the young runners will realize that running does not have to stop after high school or college, and can continue all their lives in better health than using time in unproductive ways. Some of my shirt slogans seem appropriate here such as, "LIFE IS NO DRESS REHEARSAL," "THERE IS NO FAILURE OTHER THAN IN NO LONGER TRYING," "DOING YOUR BEST IS MORE IMPORTANT THAN BEING THE BEST," "POSTERITY IS JUST AROUND THE CORNER" and "ALL'S WELL THAT ENDS WELL." Again, Amen.

Lap 80 ~ The Down Side

The negative considerations of the sport of running and jogging should be mentioned in all fairness. First as to the expense, the shoes can be expensive or not. Even the most costly are not that costly when considered the cost per mile of walking, jogging and running. A donation to a good cause for entry to a race is usually requested

The running shirts even with home lettering cost, as do different colored socks that you may have to dye yourself. Hats, gloves, cheerful colored running pants may cost as much or as little as you wish. The transportation to the race if you decide to race may be a negative factor.

For me, losing 30 pounds made my clothes hang on me so I had to purchase new clothing for my new slim figure.

My supporting wife suggested a down side was my monopolizing conversations talking about my running accomplishments at gatherings among friends.

The last negative I can think of is that a runner may have to leave a couch potato at home for an outing of jogging or running.

There is no doubt that the sport is time consuming but for any who are bored with present situations, the sport is a solution.

Since I emphasize "TAKE IT EASY," I am leaving injuries out of the negatives. As with all the warnings in my book, I could say injuries are not my fault.

In my veterinary practice, I performed as many post-mortem examinations as owners would agree to. It was astounding how black the inner-city animals' lungs were. Even without smoking, such lungs were examples of the carbon the unfortunate animals filtered from the air. So it should be mentioned that jogging or running could be the extra incentive to give up smoking. You can bank on it that carbon from tobacco smoke coating lung tissue must affect some of the areas used for oxygen absorption. Running in heavy smog areas can be a negative.

If you find other negatives jot them down and eventually let me hear about them.

Lap 81 ~ Strange as It Seems

Strange as it may seem to you and to me, too, that a retired veterinarian, sitting quietly wondering about why all dogs had Hip Dysplasia other than Greyhounds, has been led to the theory that <u>toxins</u> in foods may be incriminated as causing many conditions of ill health in dog's best friend as well as in canines.

It seems to me that the toxin or toxins work in two ways or in combination. First, by affecting the offspring through exposure while a developing fetus and, second, by slow accumulation until the toxin(s) build concentrations enough to overcome the defense system of the person, resulting in the symptoms.

It appears that some individuals may be immune to the effects of toxins and others slower to demonstrate by symptoms the damage resulting.

Then the vet takes up running and devotes hours of wonderment over why runners are healthier than non-runners. My conclusions may be subject to debate (I hope) but I have concluded that in studying and acting the part by running three or combinations of three theories are responsible for the answer to, "Why are runners healthier than non-runners?"

First, due to the increased activity of brain chemistry and, second, due to the increase of circulation of blood while running that detoxifies as it courses through the system at a greater extent than in non-runners. The Greyhounds mentioned while pregnant were trained by running to produce puppies of the speed of the mothers. (The inheritance of an acquired character-bunk.) By running, the increased circulation of blood detoxified the blood affecting the premature Greyhounds. Third, by the increase of air to the lungs eliminating dead air not eliminated while resting.

It may be that the answer to problems such as Autism could be answered by the intra-uterine theory and perhaps other conditions. Whereas conditions such as Parkinson's, ALS and elderly diabetes that starts tens of years later in runners than in non-runners, as well as many other conditions, are examples of the slow accumulation of the toxic substance(s).

The effects of people drinking water through lead plumbing all their lives and suddenly having an attack of acute lead poisoning when the daily minutia of lead accumulated becomes toxic with symptoms is well documented.

By identifying the toxin(s) if they are the cause or causes would be a major contribution to society by preventing half or more of the hospital costs in treatment and hospitalizations. More important the elimination of the problems of unknown cause(s) would prevent the sorrow of families as well as patients. The major problem lies in the need of research testing of seemingly safe food additives over the short time that can become killers when accumulated over the years. Furthermore, seemingly safe ingredients may be deadly in some percent of humans if consumed in more than a tolerable amount.

If my theory is correct that the act of running filters toxins from blood, etc., that is one answer to why runners are healthier than sedentary humans. It would seem to me that food additives or combinations may be high on a list of possibilities to study. In my lifetime, half a million metric tons or so of citric acid are added to food every year. Being harmless and perhaps desirable it does not have to appear on food labels. When tested, was it anticipated that that huge volume would be added to our food? With 30,000,000 people who run at least once a week, we have a huge number of people to compare the effects of possible toxins the general public eats regularly with the incidence of the running part.

If my considerations are valid, I repeat as mentioned in the Preface that this book could be a landmark book as was *Uncle Tom's Cabin* and *The Jungle*.

Lap 82 ~ A Personal Letter to You

Dear Senior,

Well, well, you and I have traveled many a lap together. You may have noted I tend to make light of many situations about which I should be more serious but that's only a weakness of mine. About the underlying reasons for this book, I am as serious as can be.

With study after study, the results point the way to better health as well as a longer life with real exercise and not superficial half measures. Running, taken seriously with your good judgment as to how far to go at any one time, is the best exercise I can think of. Once you agree with me, you have virtually no reason not to try it.

If you can think of no other reason to run than to prove my opinions about this sport are wrong, I will be delighted for your attempt. I personally can't think of a reason for normal seniors of any age not to start. As a senior you are well aware of the position of seniors in general in our society. Rest homes, senior condos, "out of sight out of mind" seems to be our lot, so for one of us to do something that is thought by others to be impossible seems to be against the rules. Perhaps you will wonder, "Do you suppose I could actually do it?" I am living proof that indeed it can and should be done.

Finally, this is a request from me to you. If by reading my book, *Come Jog with Me,* you have tried my recommendations and agree with me, please drop me a line or an email about your success.

Please note: We veterinarians are not permitted to write prescriptions for dog's best friend.

With love,
George Whitney

Appendix 1 ~ Physician's Consultation

These are some of the tests your doctor may call for: BUN, CL, CP2, CREATI, EGFR, GLU, K and NA for electrolytes and kidney function.

Also a BASO%, EOS, GRAN, HCT, HGB, LYMPH%, MCH, MCV, MONO%, MPV, PLT, RBC, RDW, WBC that comprise your complete blood count, your hemoglobin with a B12 and iron levels. Then comes ALP, ALT, AST, GGT and TBIL for your liver function. Next should be your CHOL, HDL, LDL, TRIG and finally your TRSH. It is amazing what a few drops of your blood can tell about your health.

Then explain that after a year of workouts and perhaps a 5k race under your belt, you would like a repeat of the tests. I predict that at that time, you will be told you no longer need heart medicine and other stuff you have been taking to prolong your life. Your doctor, be it a he or she, will likely tell you to keep on doing what you are and to check back at a later date for a follow up. With few or no problems, you may be of little interest to the human medical profession for years.

Another thought, perhaps you had better not mention that you have been referred by a veterinarian.

Appendix 2 ~ A Summary of the Program

Details of the program from walking to jogging to running

You have accepted the challenge to at least trying the program.

You have a pair of comfortable walking shoes.

Select the day of the first week you will begin your adventure.

Let's pick Mondays at 7AM.

Just walk at an interesting pace to enjoy the wonders of nature, be it in city or country. Walk until you are tired or not more than an hour.

Perhaps the first day it's for 10 minutes. GOOD! You're on your way.

Skip a day and repeat the walk and perhaps 15 minutes finds you tiring and that's OK.

Skip a day and repeat the walk perhaps for 30 minutes or until you are a little tired.

The object is to gradually walk until you are walking for an hour and feeling good about it.

Keep up the three times a week for perhaps four weeks.

Then the day has come for a second important point in your progress, the first being when you took the first step in your adventure.

This may be a good time to ask your doctor's permission to run.

This is the day when you gather your strength and step out in a jog for a few or as many paces as is comfortable for you.

Perhaps it is six short paces.

Then back to the walking until you are adventurous enough to repeat the first few jogging steps. Continue on this important day until you tire and that may be for only half an hour.

If you have come this far, you realize what is happening to you. You are feeling good in your legs and all over as you have actually started on the road to running.

Consider running shoes.

Gradually increase the jogging and the times until you tire, until you can jog without going anywhere for an hour.

At this point you don't need me to let you know that you actually feel better in your legs and generally than you have in years. That is another special point in your adventure.

Next buy a stopwatch and go out to time your progress. From a starting point jog for say 15 minutes, turn around and jog back and note the time it took you.

When you return make some notes in your log book that you have decided to keep.

The above program took me a year to think I was ready to try a 5k (3.1 miles) organized race as I report in the book.

Appendix 3 ~ Lap Art in Your Running World to Mark Up Running Shirts

Fortunately anyone can become proficient enough as an artist to letter your running shirts – even at your age – and even at mine.

Required equipment:

1. A plain white "T" shirt.
2. A marking pen of the desired color with permanent ink.
3. An ironing board or flat surface over which the shirt can be stretched. A bulletin board can do it with thumb tacks to stretch the fabric.
4. Blank paper on which to draw the quotation to size.
5. A dictionary to check your spelling for such words as METHUSELA or ONTOGONY RECAPITULATES PHYLOGENY.
6. Two straight edges to keep the marker within limits.
7. Actually sketch the quote as it should appear on the shirt, on paper.

You're all set. Cut the words on the paper in strips of the words for each line. Place the word(s) of the first line along the upper straight edge on the shirt and position them to be equal distance from each side. Place the second straight edge along the bottom of the cut out word. When centered, move the template to above the top straight edge and with a steady a hand as possible copy the wording from the paper marker to the shirt. Move the straight edges to where you will mark the second line and repeat above until the quote is complete. Here are some examples of proper spacing:

MIRROR, MIRROR
ON THE WALL
WHAT THE #@!*&#!$
HAPPENED?

SLIDING DOWN THE
RAZOR BLADE
OF
LIFE

Appendix 4 ~ Dying Socks

As far as the dying of the socks is concerned, I make a little ceremony of it because, after all, the socks will be with me through all kinds of weather and temperatures and must feel good on my feet. In my case, I think I run faster with one red and one yellow but you may have to make the final decision as to colors and composition. Most grocery stores have a good choice of colors. By the way, start with comfortable white socks of your preferred length and size. Coordinate your shirt colors with your socks, or not, it's up to you. And remember "TIE."

Appendix 5 ~ Prejudice Letter

Race Director or Race Committee Chairman or whatever

Dear --------,

In your application for your 5k race on such and such a date. I note the top age group as 60 and up. That is an unacceptable example of prejudice and has been eliminated for most races. We older-age runners object and have agreed to boycott all races with such restrictions. Perhaps you will correct that blunder for next year's race and recognize all age groups as the USATF does.

Sincerely,

XXXXX

Appendix 6 ~ Running Shirt Slogans Used So Far by the Author

- OXYGEN IS OVERRATED
- CALL 911
- ALWAYS BEING RIGHT IS AN AWFUL RESPONSIBILITY
- MOTHER TOLD ME NEVER TO ASSOCIATE WITH FAST WOMEN
- HAVE YOU GOT AN EXTRA CIGARETTE?
- THE LUNATICS ARE IN CHARGE OF THE ASYLUM
- RUN LIKE YOU STOLE SOMETHING
- IF I WERE A HORSE, THEY'D SHOOT ME
- DON'T RUN IN MY FOOTSTEPS, I THINK I STEPPED IN SOMETHING
- SPOILED ROTTEN HUSBAND
- PASSING PERMITTED
- RUNNING FROM THE UNDERTAKER
- THOSE WHO EXERCISE DIE HEALTHIER
- FEEL BLUE? START BREATHING AGAIN
- BEWARE OF ALLIGATORS
- USE TACT, FATHEAD
- RUN LIKE A SNAKE IS GAINING
- EVER TRY HITCHHIKING?
- YOU DON'T HAVE TO BE CRAZY TO RUN BUT IT HELPS
- METHUSELAH
- OH, TO BE 84 AGAIN (or whatever)

- IT'S LONELY BACK HERE
- ONTOGENY RECAPITULATES PHYLOGENY
- HALFFAST
- WHEN CLINTON LIED NOBODY DIED
- I'M NO MARION JONES
- I'M NO CHRIS DICKERSON
- FASTER. MARTY SCHAIVONE IS GAINING ON US
- I'M MUCH TOO YOUNG TO BE THIS OLD
- I INTEND TO RUN FOREVER. SO FAR SO GOOD.
- WHAT ONE RELISHES NOURISHES
- IF YOU'RE BEHIND ME, YOU BETTER BE ANCIENT
- I DON'T SUFFER FROM INSANITY, I ENJOY IT
- AGE ISN'T IMPORTANT UNLESS YOU'RE CHEESE
- SLIDING DOWN THE RAZOR BLADE OF LIFE
- BIRDS GOTTA FLY, FISH GOTTA SWIM
- GROWING UP IS MANDATORY, GROWING OLD IS OPTIONAL
- POSTERITY IS JUST AROUND THE CORNER
- NOT ON STEROIDS (yet)
- NOT ON STEROIDS BUT THANKS FOR ASKING
- NEVER TRUST A NAKED RUNNER
- NEVER TRUST A NAKED MALE RUNNER
- MIRROR, MIRROR ON THE WALL, WHAT THE +##&*!# HAPPENED?
- JESUS IS COMING – LOOK BUSY

- OLD AGE IS NATURE'S SENSE OF HUMOR
- EXCUSE MY DUST
- FAST AS A HOG ON ICE
- IT JUST LOOKS EASY
- BE THE CHANGE YOU WANT TO SEE
- FASTER THAN SOME TURTLES
- IF I'D KNOWN I WOULD LIVE THIS LONG, I'D HAVE TAKEN BETTER CARE OF ME
- A RETIRED HUSBAND IS A WIFE'S FULL-TIME JOB
- LOOK BEFORE OR YOU'LL FIND YOURSELF BEHIND
- I'M A LITTLE BEHIND
- OLD AGE ISN'T BAD IF YOU CONSIDER THE ALTERNATIVE
- NOTHING IS SO FIRMLY BELIEVED AS WHAT WE LEAST KNOW
- NEARLY ALL DIE OF THEIR REMEDIES – NOT THEIR ILLNESSES
- ASPIRATION, INSPIRATION, DEDICATION, PERSPIRATION
- S/HE WHO LAUGHS, LASTS
- I FEEL LIKE A MILLION – EVERY YEAR OF IT
- I NEED A CHECK UP FROM THE NECK UP
- I'M SHORT ON HORSE POWER AND LONG ON EXHAUST
- WE'RE MAKING MORE ENEMIES THAN WE'RE KILLING
- LIFE IS A TERMINAL DISEASE

- SO FAR THIS IS THE OLDEST I'VE BEEN
- HUNTERS SHOULD EAT WHAT THEY SHOOT
- ONE NATION UNDER SURVEILLANCE
- LUCK? NO. IT'S SKILL AND GUTS
- NOT RUNNING FOR SEVEN DAYS MAKES ONE WEAK
- IMAGINATION IS MORE IMPORTANT THAN KNOWLEDGE
- BIBAMUS MORIENDUM EST. DEATH'S UNAVOIDABLE
- NEVER TRUST A NAKED GORILLA
- RUNNING FROM THE BILL COLLECTOR
- SUPPORT BACTERIA. THEY'RE THE ONLY CULTURE SOME PEOPLE HAVE
- ON THE OTHER HAND – YOU HAVE DIFFERENT FINGERS
- LOST IN THOUGHT – UNFAMILIAR TERRITORY
- A DAY WITHOUT SUNSHINE IS LIKE – NIGHT
- HE WHO LAUGHS LAST THINKS SLOWEST
- I DRIVE WAY TOO FAST TO WORRY ABOUT CHOLESTEROL
- HALF THE PEOPLE YOU KNOW ARE BELOW AVERAGE
- THE OLDER THE FIDDLE, THE SWEETER THE TUNE
- I FORGOT WHY I'M HERE
- THE FURTURE IS NOT WHAT IT USED TO BE
- LIFE LIVED FOR TOMORROW WILL ALWAYS BE A DAY AWAY
- IF I WERE A BUILDING THEY'D DEMOLISH ME

- BORN AGAIN RUNNER

- LITERACY AIN'T EVERYTHING

- THOSE WHO STAND FOR NOTHING FALL FOR EVERYTHING

- KEEP OFF GRASS

- DOING YOUR BEST IS MORE IMPORTANT THAN BEING THE BEST

- 3 THINGS I FORGET. NAMES, FACES AND THE OTHER I CAN'T REMEMBER

- RETIREMENT CAN BE FATAL

- ME TARZAN, YOU JANE?

- THERE IS NO FAILURE EXCEPT IN NO LONGER TRYING

- I'M CONFUSED. WAIT, MAYBE I'M NOT

- I KNOW I CAME HERE FOR SOMETHING

- WHICH WOULD YOU RATHER DO OR GO RUNNING?

- DOES THE NAME PAVLOV RING A BELL?

- WHY DID GOD GIVE ADAM AND EVE NAVELS?

- HOORAY FOR ORIGINAL SIN

- THE COST OF LIVING HAS GONE UP A DOLLAR A BOTTLE

- SUCCESS IS A JOURNEY, NOT A DESTINATION

- INSANITY IS HEREDITARY. YOU GET IT FROM YOUR CHILDREN

- IN TIME OF WAR THE FIRST CAUSALITY IS TRUTH

- THERE ARE NO WARLIKE PEOPLE. ONLY WARLIKE LEADERS

- TEACH! DON'T PREACH IN PUBLIC SCHOOLS
- THE WAR WOULD END IF THE DEAD RETURNED
- ALL'S WELL THAT ENDS WELL
- SLOW AND STEADY WILL NOT WIN THIS RACE
- I'M IN TRAINING FOR RETIREMENT
- HANG IN THERE
- YOU COULD BE HOME WATCHING TV
- SMILE OR AT LEAST SMIRK
- FOLLOW ME AND YOU'LL BE LATE
- DO UNTO OTHERS BEFORE THEY DO UNTO YOU
- DO UNTO OTHERS AS THEY WOULD BE DONE UNTO
- WHEN BEFRIENDED REMEMBER IT. WHEN YOU BEFRIEND, FORGET IT
- WHO PLEASURE GIVES SHALL JOY RECEIVE
- WOULD YOU PERSUADE, SPEAK OF INTEREST, NOT OF REASON
- NECESSITY NEVER MADE A GOOD BARGAIN
- WELL DONE IS BETTER THAN WELL SAID
- NOT ALL WHO RUN ARE LOST
- NEVER TAKE LIFE SERIOUSLY. NOBODY GETS OUT OF IT ALIVE
- IF IT'S TO BE IT'S UP TO ME
- A WINNER NEVER QUITS. A QUITTER NEVER WINS
- HONK IF YOU LOVE PEACE AND QUIET

- THE EARLY BIRD GETS THE WORM BUT THE SECOND MOUSE GETS THE CHEESE
- ANYONE WHO HATES CHILDREN AND DOGS CAN'T BE ALL BAD
- WHEN THE POWER OF LOVE OVERCOMES THE LOVE OF POWER WE WILL HAVE PEACE
- INTELLIGENT DESIGN, THE EVOLUTION OF IGNORANCE
- WHY IS THERE MONEY FOR WAR AND NOT FOR EDUCATION?

Appendix 7 ~ Substitute with Running

In checking out some ads and articles in two magazines I note that there is advice on all sorts of medication and stuff for human welfare most of which is expensive. With the word, "running" in place of the stuff, it makes sense and would cost almost nothing.

Here are a few examples:

- You don't have to hike the John Muir Trail, you can run it.
- Nine out of 10 cardiologists endorse running.
- Running can help stress, joint pain, back pain, poor circulation, insomnia, high blood pressure, headaches and corns.
- Running can increase mobility.
- Running can increase blood circulation.
- Running can energize the body.
- One small step and you can start running.
- Your jogging adventure continues long after the run ends.
- With running you are part of the solution to good health.
- Make your running adventure unforgettable.
- River running. 10 days of wilderness wonder.

- Running is easy on you and the environment.

- Running is a great escape.

- Nothing clears the mind like a change of scenery. *Come Jog with Me.*

- In running you can make a difference.

- The finest running this side of Bangkok.

- Expertise, knowledge and advice is available at no extra charge at your local running store. Tell them I sent you.

- Don't be fooled by imitations.

Check it out for yourself. Such information is available in many magazines if you substitute the word "running" for the subject of the ads.

Appendix 8 ~ All American USATF Times

Road Running Standards of Excellence
for Men for a 5k Race

60-64	24:43
65-69	25:53
70-74	27:40
75-79	29:48
80-84	33:34
85-89	39:37
90-94	50:21
95+	1:13:11

Road Running Standards of Excellence
for Women for a 5k Race

60-64	30:09
65-69	32:32
70-74	35:20
75-79	38:38
80-84	43:05
85-89	51:47
90-94	1:11:05
95+	2:13:29

Appendix 9 ~ Contacts

When your fingers wander idly over the computer keys (as the song goes) perhaps you will look into what the other half of runners is concerned with. Here are some contacts at random for you to check out. Many are magazines. Perhaps some are in your area. This is a partial list.

- American College of Sports Medicine (All)
- American Journal of Preventive Medicine
- American Medical Athletic Association (All)
- American Running Association
- American Track and Field (CA)
- Athletics Magazine (Canada/All)
- Austin Runner
- California Track News
- Canadian Running Magazine
- Chicago Runner
- Christine Luff
- Club Running (Mag)
- Club Running (network)
- Cool Running
- Eastern Track
- Exchange Zone (USATF NE)
- Fast Forward (USATF)
- Fastracks (All)
- Florida Running

- Georgia Runner
- Hitekracing.com (CT)
- Inside Alabama Track
- Inside Texas Running Magazine
- International Society for Anthropology
- JBsports.com (CT)
- Keeping Track (OR)
- Long Island Footnotes
- Michigan Runner
- Midwest Runner
- Missouri Runner and Triathlete
- National Masters News (US)
- New England Over 65 Runners Club (NE)
- New England Runner (NE)
- New Jersey Track
- Northwest Runner
- NTSSAW (NY)
- Racing South (SE)
- Rails to Trails Conservancy (US)
- Run Minnesota
- Runner (NJ & CT)
- Runner's gazette (Mid Atlantic)
- Runners World (All)
- Running and Fitness News (Americanrunning.org)
- Running Journal (SE)

- Running Med News
- Running Network, LLC Box 801, Fort Anderson, WI 53538
- Running News (NY)
- Running Research News (MI)
- Running Times (All)
- Running, Ranting, Racing (MD)
- Southern Track and Field News (SC et el)
- Sprintic Magazine
- Sweat Magazine (AZ)
- TAFWA News (CA)
- The Runner Magazine
- The Winged Foot (NTC)
- Track and Field News (US)
- Track and Field Stats (CA)
- Track Newsletter (CA)
- Track South Journal (VA to FL)
- Trackwire (All)
- Trackwire for Women (All)
- Trail Runner Magazine (CO)
- Ultra Running
- USA Track and Field
- USATF (US)
- Washington Running Report (E)

Appendix 10 ~ Poetry

Good Life

On the various paths of good life
Are well hidden wastes not overt to strife
For hidden wastes gather days and nights
Unknown to all of the eventual plights

'Till wastes add up to less happy days
As slowly our life is passing its ways.
The cause of the ageing defies all wealth
As the wastes are reaching insurmountable health.

There are ways to dispel the gathering storm
So listen to me and don't be forlorn
With the wastes that are in us day and night.
To do it is no mysterious fight.

Just make up your mind to have a good fling
At actually running or some other thing
To flush the innards with all your might
And lo and behold most waste will take flight.

And with a new life you are free to behold
New vigorous days as of days of old.

Others Try

Some thinking humans run
Past childhood days just for fun.
Please someone tell me why
Some don't and others try.

All people born can think
From knowledge all too many slink.
Please someone tell me why
Some don't and others try.

Since runners are the best of health
And measure health as part of wealth
Please someone tell me why
Some don't and others try.

Some runners are thinkers too
And thrive in sun and rain and dew
I'm someone here to tell you why,
The thinkers learned enough to try.

Do Unto Others as They Would Be Done Unto

We know the reason for life to be present
As one form existing for leader and peasant.
Other creatures seem born to be used
In view of the many who choose to abuse.

But what is the fight for some to use might
Regardless of feelings of those who have right
When reason is sung by those who don't care
To the tune of profit with pain unaware?

For eons of time has created each creature.
To marvel at action and structure of feature
To think of the charm that one would be
Both here and now for us to see.

Respect all life for you who read
It's wrong for any to inflict pain by deed
On wild life, game part of life's treasure.
Stand and protest man's evil called pleasure.

And strain to awaken love, caring, adore
All living things treat with kindness and more
Please don't do to others be they man or beast
What they would not choose you to do in the least.

The Sun is Rising

The sun is rising in the sky
For me to tell the reason why
A fuller day waits your wealth
It comes to you as better health

For those whose age has cast its spell
This news has come to wish you well
To show you all new thoughts sublime
To add you years of better time.

All know of worthy goals to find
Require time and thought of mind
So start today with all your might
To get in shape to be just right.

It means a change of ways and deeds
To grant your body all it needs
For better metabolic function
Facing many at this junction.

Dispel the wastes that come with ages
Relearning running as your wages
For all who say it can't be done
To follow you with having fun.

Still they fail to wish you well then
Tell them all to go to pell mell again.
The trick is to rid the body by way of running
What couldn't be done by sitting and sunning.

Before the sun descends the sky
Plan to join with all to try.
The prize to you for all to access
Is wealth with health and happiness.

When Wealth is Health

A child I ran as any kid.
A teen I ran as others did.
To run was never on any list.
To work was high up to resist.

Through life I rested my aging way
Not trying labor as others may.
Til all my vim and vigor had parted
Twas then by need my wits had started

To find the road to regain my health
A thought of value more than wealth.
The road was running as trial for me
But would my years of rest agree?

Indeed they did and I'm here to say
I've learned a lot along the way
From walking and jogging for many a try
With wonder and ponder and always a why?

Why feel better than past recent years
With miles left behind as part of the cheers
With less loss of breath on climbing a stair
And stronger legs my weight to bear.

I think I have found a secret sublime
Of life as close to the fountain of time
In running and only are we internally geared
To rid inner circles of stuff to be feared.

Now you know for all to tell
Why learning to run will make a spell
Of better days with better wealth
That comes to runners as better health.

11/21/10

Made in the USA
Lexington, KY
22 March 2012